D1388560

coping and thriving in
nursing

an essential guide to practice

peter j. martin

Cavell Nurses' Trust

When nurses suffer hardship, Cavell Nurses' Trust gives help. We're #HereFor Nurses.

Cavell Nurses' Trust supports UK nurses, midwives and healthcare assistants, both working and retired, when they're suffering personal or financial hardship, often due to illness, disability, older age and domestic abuse. The nurses, midwives and healthcare assistants we help say that they're often happier, healthier and able to stay in or return to work.

From simple, essential support like money to repairing a broken cooker or boiler, to vital life-changing aid like helping a family flee their home due to domestic abuse, Cavell Nurses' Trust is here to help. We're a charity and we help people at no cost to themselves.

Nurses are the vital backbone of our healthcare system, doing difficult work under great pressure for the benefit of us all. We were shocked to find that nursing professionals are twice as likely as the public to suffer financial hardship. Worryingly, they are also three times as likely to suffer domestic abuse. This is appalling and we're taking action.

We rely on our generous supporters and fantastic fundraisers, individuals, community groups and organisations, to fund the help we give to nurses suffering hardship. Without these people, the charity would not exist. We want to see a society that cares for the people that care for it. There are many ways you can show your support and be #HereForNurses, from fundraising to making a donation.

Thank you to Peter, Mary, Cathy, Steve, Martin, Tess, Ness and Caroline for choosing to help Cavell Nurses' Trust through making a donation from every copy of *Coping and Thriving in Nursing* sold.

For more information, please visit: www.cavellnursestrust.org

Or get in touch at: admin@cavellnursestrust.org or 01527 595 999.

coping and thriving in
nursing
an essential guide to practice
peter j. martin

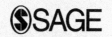

Los Angeles | London | New Delhi
Singapore | Washington DC | Melbourne

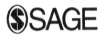

Los Angeles | London | New Delhi
Singapore | Washington DC | Melbourne

SAGE Publications Ltd
1 Oliver's Yard
55 City Road
London EC1Y 1SP

SAGE Publications Inc.
2455 Teller Road
Thousand Oaks, California 91320

SAGE Publications India Pvt Ltd
B 1/I 1 Mohan Cooperative Industrial Area
Mathura Road
New Delhi 110 044

SAGE Publications Asia-Pacific Pte Ltd
3 Church Street
#10-04 Samsung Hub
Singapore 049483

Editor: Alex Clabburn
Editorial assistant: Jade Grogan
Production editor: Katie Forsythe
Proofreader: Bryan Campbell
Indexer: Gary Kirby
Marketing manager: Tamara Navaratnam
Cover design: Wendy Scott
Typeset by: C&M Digitals (P) Ltd, Chennai, India
Printed in the UK
Editorial arrangement, Introduction and Editorial

Editorial arrangement, Introduction and
Conclusion © Peter J. Martin 2018

Chapters 1 and 8 © Mary Kennedy 2018
Chapters 2 and 6 © Steve Wood 2018
Chapters 3 © Peter J. Martin and Martin Harrison 2018
Chapters 4 and 10 © Cathy Constable 2018
Chapter 5 © Caroline Barratt and Tess Wagstaffe 2018
Chapter 7 © Tess Wagstaffe and Ness
   Woodcock-Dennis 2018
Chapter 9 © Martin Harrison and Peter J. Martin 2018

First published 2018

Library of Congress Control Number: 2018931917

British Library Cataloguing in Publication data

A catalogue record for this book is available from the
British Library

ISBN 978-1-5264-2360-3
ISBN 978-1-5264-2361-0 (pbk)

At SAGE we take sustainability seriously. Most of our products are printed in the UK using responsibly sourced
papers and boards. When we print overseas we ensure sustainable papers are used as measured by the
PREPS grading system. We undertake an annual audit to monitor our sustainability.

Contents

About the Editor and Contributors

Caroline Barratt (MRes, PhD) is a lecturer at the School of Health and Social Care at the University of Essex and has wide-ranging academic and research experience. Her main interests are in mental health, social inequality, qualitative research methodologies and contemplative pedagogy. She is particularly passionate about the integration of contemplative practice in higher education, not only as a means of improving student performance and resilience but also of transforming how they relate to themselves, the world and one another and of building the foundations of meaningful social change. She established the Contemplative Pedagogy Network (www.contemplativepedagogynetwork.com) in 2014, and developed a course for health and social care professionals entitled 'Mindfulness, Self-Compassion and Compassionate Care', in which contemplative practice is embedded. She has published in a variety of academic journals and books, including an article on mindfulness and self-compassion for nurses in the *Nursing Standard* and has been invited to speak at European events on mindfulness in education. Having first learnt to meditate in 2000, Caroline is a trained Mindfulness-Based Stress Reduction (MBRS) teacher and attends several meditation retreats each year.

Cathy Constable (MA, RGN, RMN, SFHEA) qualified as an RGN in 1988 and went on to qualify as an RMN in 1991. Cathy worked in clinical practice as a mental health nurse for 20 years, across inpatient and community settings. She also worked for Colchester Mind and was instrumental in developing and managing a community-based early intervention service for young people with emotional and behavioural issues. During this time, Cathy was involved in national research on social inclusion of hard-to-reach young people with the Mental Health Foundation and the Social Inclusion Unit.

Since 2010, Cathy has worked as a Mental Health lecturer at the University of Essex and is Programme Lead for the Nursing Mental Health (pre-registration) programme. She is a Senior Fellow of the Higher Education Academy, and has an MA in Psychoanalytical Studies and is interested in Child and Adolescent mental health issues, working with service users with acute and ongoing mental health issues and organisational dynamics.

Martin Harrison (MSc, DipN, RMN, PGDip Med & Clin Education) is Professional Lead for Mental Health Nursing at the University of Essex. Martin's background is in mental health nursing; he qualified 30 years ago and has worked in practice, management and education.

Martin has a particular interest in substance misuse services. In Wales, Martin designed and delivered the first NHS syringe exchange scheme, working with a rural population living in remote communities. In addition, he has also been active in promoting service user involvement and health research ethics.

Martin gained an MSc in Nursing in 1995 and subsequently qualified as a nurse teacher in 2010. He has worked at the University of Essex since 2004, joining it at the inception of the MSc Nursing pre-registration programme. For eight years, he was the Programme Lead for the MS Nursing Mental Health (pre-registration) programme.

Mary Kennedy (MSc, PhD in Nursing, RN (Adult), RN (Mental Health), RN (General), DMS, Diploma in Counselling, FAETC), is a mental health nurse and worked in the NHS for nearly 40 years. She held a variety of nursing roles before leaving the NHS in 2016, and has since joined the University of Essex as a Mental Health lecturer.

Mary has a wide range of clinical, research and academic experience and in leading service development and innovation within clinical practice. She has published reports and articles on a range of subjects and co-authored a chapter on vulnerable groups in mental health. Her specific interest is dementia care and in developing services to improve the delivery of care for people with dementia and their families. Within the university, Mary has led on the development of dementia education for health and social care practitioners working in the NHS and the private sector.

She is particularly interested in the delivery of compassionate care and trained at the 'Point of Care Foundation' to deliver and facilitate Schwartz Rounds in the NHS to help improve patients' experience of care and increase support for the staff who work in healthcare. She is now involved in developing this initiative within higher education.

Peter J. Martin (RMN, DipN, BN, CertEd(FE), RNT PhD (Wales)) qualified as a mental health nurse in 1983 and worked in practice, management and education roles within mental health services. Currently, Peter is at the University of Essex, where he is Director of Education and Professor at the School of Health and Social Care. In 2001, he developed the university's Professional Doctorate in Health and Social Care programme, which he continues to lead.

Amongst other publications, Peter has co-authored with Mark Fox and Gill Green the book, *Doing Practitioner Research* (London: Sage, 2007); and co-edited with Kimmy Eldridge the book, *Partnerships in Healthcare* (London: Quay Books, 2006).

Tess Wagstaffe (MA, DipN, RMN, RT, FHEA) is a mental health lecturer at the University of Essex and has worked in clinical practice as a mental health nurse for over 20 years in Adult Acute Mental Health and Child and Adolescent Mental Health Services. Tess has an MA in Sociology and the Psychodynamics of Mental Health. Her interests include deliberate self-harm and suicide risk assessment, having worked in liaison with the local A&E department, conducting out-of-hours assessments and also being involved in the formation of 'out-of-hours' mental health services.

Tess's research for her Master's degree involved interviewing nurses and exploring their experiences of working with deliberate self-harm in the community and inpatient settings. Currently teaching nursing at MSc and BSc level, Tess is involved in exploring student experience of equality in the university and clinical placement areas.

Steve Wood (MA, BSc (Hons), PGCE, RNT, DipN, RMN, RGN) is a Mental Health lecturer at the University of Essex and has wide-ranging academic, research and nursing practice experience. His specialist interest is person-centred dementia care and he has published a number of papers, reports and book chapters on this subject. These include supporting family carers, evaluating a memory service and applying the VERA communication framework. Steve is currently undertaking a participatory action research study that involves the use of life-story work in an age-inclusive dementia service. He has also undertaken research that explores the learning and professional socialisation experiences of mental health student nurses.

Ness Woodcock-Dennis (Dip HE RN (Adult), SCPHN (RHV), PG Dip MaCE (RNT), SfHEA, FRSPH) is an adult nurse and Specialist Community Public Health Nurse. She has worked in a surgical environment and in Children's Services as a sexual health and family planning practitioner, in addition to working as a health visitor, nurse prescriber and community practice teacher.

As an experienced Health Visitor working in child protection situations, Ness is specifically interested in the concepts of compassion fatigue and practitioner burnout and the need to create a compassionate culture within organisations to support practitioners. She is currently Nursing Lecturer and Module Lead at the University of Essex for Delivering Compassionate Care as an Adult Nurse.

Acknowledgements

Reviewers

We would like to thank the students and lecturers who helped to review this book's content, providing valuable feedback to shape an important book for student nurses and practitioners. These include the following:

Susan Barker, Cardiff University

Steven Trenoweth, Bournemouth University

Ann Felton, University of Nottingham

Iris Gault, Kingston University

Publisher's Acknowledgements

The authors and publisher are grateful to the relevant third parties for their kind permission to reproduce the following material:

Extract from World Health Organization (2010) *Healthy Workplaces: A Model for Action for Employers. For Employers, Workers, Policy-makers and Practitioners*. Geneva: World Health Organization.

Reference to Schwartz Rounds® in Chapter 1, an organisation that provides staff with a safe and facilitated space to discuss the emotional and social aspects of working in healthcare. Created by The Schwartz Center for Compassionate Healthcare® in Boston, MA.

Banja's five principles, Banja, J. (2010) 'The normalization of deviance in healthcare delivery', *Business Horizons*, 53: 139–148. Reproduced with permission of Elsevier.

Value Functions bullet point list, Pattison, S., and Thomas B., (2010) 'Healthcare professions and their changing values: pulling professions together', in S. Pattison, B. Hannigan, R. Pill and B. Thomas (eds) (2010) *Emerging Values in Healthcare*. London: Jessica Kingsley Publishers.

Extract from Woodbridge, K. and Fulford, B. (2005) *Whose Values? A Workbook for Values-Based Practice in Mental Health Care*. London: Sainsbury Centre for Mental Health. Now named the Centre for Mental Health.

Extract from Schön, D.A. (1987) *Educating the Reflective Practitioner: Toward a New Design for Teaching and Learning in the Professions*. San Francisco, CA: Jossey-Bass. Reproduced with permission of John Wiley and Sons.

Figure 7.1 The components of compassion, Neff, K. (2003) 'Self-compassion: An alternative conceptualization of a healthy attitude toward oneself', *Self and Identity*, 2: 85–101. Reproduced with permission of Taylor & Francis.

Figure 8.2: Arnstein's Ladder of Participation (1969), Arnstein, S.R. (1969) 'A ladder of citizen participation', *Journal of the American Planning Association*, 35: 216–224. Reproduced with permission of Taylor & Francis.

Box 10.1: Indications of positive and negative transference and counter transference in nursing relationships, Jones, A. (2005) 'Transference, counter-transference and repetition: Some implications for nursing practice', *Journal of Clinical Nursing*, 14: 1177–1184. Reproduced with permission of John Wiley and Sons.

Activity 10.1: Reflective exercise on family origins, Senge, P.M. (1999) *The Dance of Change: The Challenges of Sustaining Momentum in Learning Organizations*. New York: Currency/Doubleday.

Box 10.5 The value and therapeutic benefit of writing, Johns, C. and Johns, C. (2017) *Becoming A Reflective Practitioner*. Hoboken, NJ: Wiley-Blackwell. Reproduced with permission of John Wiley and Sons.

Introduction

Talking to Nurses

Peter J. Martin

As a nurse lecturer, I spend a lot of time with nurses and, consequently, spend a lot of time also talking about nursing to those who deliver nursing care to people. These conversations are with students who see one facet of the nursing environment and with qualified nurses who often see a very different facet.

Students talk about the community of practice (Lave and Wenger, 1991) that they are seeking to enter, and this conversation is often about their own anxieties about being 'good enough' to do the job. Qualified nurses talk about the reality of their practice and their desire to do a good, personally satisfying job in an environment that sometimes seems to conspire against this goal.

In such conversations with nurses, I am particularly interested in the words and phrases that are used and in the pervading tone that underpins such accounts from practice. These descriptions of practice say a lot about how nurses are experiencing practice today.

I want to begin by recounting a short story to act as an exemplar for all of these conversations. I have brought together a number of similar accounts from different people and given them the voice of a single person. For the purposes of this story, the conversation was with a critical care adult nurse called Cleo.

Cleo worked in a critical care unit in an acute care trust at a local general hospital. She was at a stage in her career when she was thinking about undertaking a course of academic study at my university, and we were looking at what might be appropriate to her own needs and those of her workplace.

Cleo is a highly professional practitioner, with more than two decades of experience. As is often the case when nurses get together, our academic consultation turned into a conversation. We agreed that the healthcare system in which we had both trained many years ago was now very different; there had always been pressures and stresses in nursing based on the emotional labour (Hochschild, 1983) that is part of the job. However, in the early twenty-first century, these pressures do appear to be increasing, and are added to by the demographic changes in the United Kingdom, a tough economic climate and a changing professional relationship between nurses and patients.

Cleo began to describe a recent incident, where one of her staff had been involved in a medication error. The incident was undoubtedly complex but, listening to Cleo, I became more and more aware that other issues were being drawn into her story. This fairly minor incident, where no one was harmed, had become the catalyst for lifting the lid on Pandora's box, in which were contained all the problems of the UK healthcare system. Out of the Pandora's box flew a vast array of major and minor issues, all of which were having an impact on Cleo and which became incorporated into her tale. Importantly, these were issues over which Cleo felt that she had, as an individual, minimal control. In the telling of the tale, incompetent 'management', the Nursing and Midwifery Council (NMC), poor ward staffing levels and the rights and wrongs of nursing practice, to name but a few, were incorporated.

Cleo's outpouring of problems was troubling enough. But, perhaps more worrying, was that what had started as a conversation, very quickly became Cleo's own monologue. As the incident being described became increasingly inclusive of Cleo's many other concerns, my role became simply to listen and respond non-verbally at suitable places. As a mental health nurse talking to an acute care nurse, my knowledge of the detail of what was being described was, at best, scanty. Some of the conditions, interventions and clinical test readings were outside of my knowledge base, but this didn't seem to matter to Cleo; she had begun her tale and was going to recount it in her way until the end was reached.

My professional background as a mental health nurse came to the fore and I disengaged from the clinical detail of the story, my role had become insignificant, anyway. I tried to understand what was really going on for Cleo. I wondered whether this story had been told before, where it had been rehearsed. But, primarily, I wondered if it had been recounted to anyone who understood the complex details or to someone who was in a position to do anything about the direness of the situation that Cleo described. I wondered if this was one story on which Cleo had been ruminating or was this just a single exemplar of everyday practice. If this was just one of many stories on which Cleo was constantly ruminating, then how was she able to function effectively in her workplace? The respect that Cleo's colleagues had for her indicated that she was certainly able to perform her role to a very high standard; so, maybe, this was just 'muzac' in the back of Cleo's mind that accompanied her day.

An image of Cleo standing on a beach trying to hold back the tide but slowly getting overwhelmed came into my mind. Simultaneously, I thought about the sea walls, flood defence zones, life jackets and lifeboats, all tools that might help to ease the situation. I was aware that there were many tools available to help Cleo survive the everyday pressures under which she was working. Such tools may help to prevent people getting burnt out, leaving nursing or developing an increasing indifference and callousness to the suffering of others.

A few days later, I shared my experience of listening to Cleo with some of the colleagues with whom I work. I talked about my own compassionate response when listening to Cleo's tale, but also of my distress at the apparent absence of any structured support for Cleo in the workplace. I acknowledged that there may already be policies and procedures in the hospital in which Cleo worked that she was unwilling or unable to engage; but, nonetheless, she remained someone in urgent need of constructive supervision.

Each one of my colleagues present at this informal meeting recounted similar tales of emotionally draining discussions with practice colleagues. All of us recognised that the level of anxiety routinely carried by practitioners was something that we needed to address honestly in preparing students for practice. We recognised also that this needed to be embedded throughout the nursing programme and not just added on in the final study module. It was from this discussion that our response of 'Coping and Thriving in Nursing' began to emerge.

What Do We Mean by 'Coping and Thriving'?

The people who have contributed chapters to this book all work as nurse educators at the University of Essex. We work with various students of health and social care, and also with qualified practitioners who are either returning to study or contributing to our programmes as specialists. We have called this book *Coping and Thriving in Nursing* – a title that emerged through its writing.

We have tried throughout to give an honest account of practice as it is currently presented by those to whom we talk. We saw no value in presenting a fairy-tale image of health and social care; this would have been disingenuous to our practice colleagues. We wanted to acknowledge that, in our experience, there were many nurses in distress and that there were ways in which that distress could be reduced.

Nurses come into nursing because of a desire to care for others who are experiencing health or social-care-related needs: we were keen not to lose sight of this principle. Our initial title used the word 'surviving' but, whilst retaining a realistic portrayal of practice, we wanted to highlight that nurses can do more than survive, they can cope and thrive. If nurses are coping and thriving, then they can discover or rediscover the satisfaction that led them into the job in the first place.

If nurses discover or rediscover that satisfaction with their work, then they are in a much stronger position to help people find a sense of hope in illness and adversity.

Is This Book for You?

There are the 'swampy lowlands of practice' and the 'high solid grounds of academia' (Schön, 1983: 43). In the swampy lowlands, there are complex, real-world problems, for which there are no simple answers; it is a world of uncertainty, instability and value judgements. In the high grounds of academia, there is less complexity, problems are clearer and more straightforward; there are many fewer value judgements. So, if you are already a qualified practitioner and find yourself wondering what we, as educators, have to offer you, as a practitioner, it is understandable.

Our concern is the preparation of nurses to enter the workforce. In this role, we want to ensure that students leaving our programmes are highly skilled, knowledgeable, compassionate and resilient. The current standards for pre-registration nurse education (NMC, 2010) are explicit that Higher Education Institutions share this role equally with Practice Partners. It is, therefore, a legitimate concern for nurse educators when the Nursing and Midwifery Council observe that practice placement quality and capacity continues to pose a challenge to student learning (2017).

We want our students to have a good practice experience and to learn the necessary skills of coping in a contemporary health and social care system. These two points are not one and the same. We have had students who have learned nursing practice from brilliant practitioners, from people who have such skill and compassion.

Days later, we hear that the same person has left nursing or gone on long-term sick leave through stress. We want to prepare nurses for practice, in which they can cope and thrive and not be driven rapidly into leaving the profession.

So, whilst we cannot solve the problems of practice, we can, at least, offer some ways of managing and working with these problems.

Whilst the title of the book is *Coping and Thriving in Nursing*, the contents will resonate with any health and social care practitioner. The issues and problems described in relation to nursing practice will be experienced by all of the other professional groups within the health and social care sector.

We hope that health and social care students will find an introduction to the complex problems of practice alongside strategies for 'getting through', without being personally damaged by the experience. We also hope that health and social care practitioners will recognise practice-based scenarios and have a chance to consider what actions they took in similar circumstance and to learn new strategies that they can employ within their everyday practice.

Whatever the background or position, all readers will find tools and techniques underpinned by published work that seek to help us understand and survive working in emotionally demanding and complex organisations.

I regularly use my local health and social care services and generally get good quality care. On occasions, it has been suboptimal, a practitioner has been a tad offhand, an appointment postponed or a message poorly communicated. At other times, the service that I received has been exemplary, compassionate, knowledgeable, skilled and sensitive, justifying a letter to the Trust's Chief Executive Officer. Such examples, both of excellence and of averageness, are, in reality, exceptions; most times, it is 'good enough', leaving me with a sense of having received satisfactory care.

There is clearly good quality nursing care occurring every single day in our health and social services. Don't get me wrong, I don't mind a little aspiration 'to be the best'; but I am concerned about how realistic it is, striving to be the best, given the available resources in the UK National Health Service funding system. How much damage do we do to good, caring people, who, for reasons often outside of their control, are not 'the best' but who are eminently satisfactory? Maybe, we all need to be reminded occasionally that, without the 'people', we would have no health service.

We hope that you will find something in this book that helps you get through today and future days:

- If you are a *health or social care practitioner* who is finding the work environment challenging and stressful, then, in this book, we hope that you will find skills and techniques that will help you rediscover why you came into such an emotionally demanding job in the first place.
- If you are a *health or social care student* preparing to enter practice, then we hope that you will find in these pages the skills and techniques to enable you to be an excellent practitioner, who recognises the importance of their own well-being and takes steps to protect it.
- If you are a *health and social care manager*, then we hope that, in these pages, you will find strategies and techniques that you can share with your team to enable them to be excellent practitioners, who have the resilience to manage daily in the emotionally complex world of health and social care.

Chapters

The chapters in this book are all self-contained and each author presents their own perspective on the general theme of coping and thriving. As such, each chapter represents a discrete essay on a topic relevant to surviving in contemporary health and social care services.

In addition, each chapter can be seen as offering a different facet of coping and thriving, from which a series of common themes begin to emerge. These themes are summarised and presented as a toolkit in the final chapter.

In Chapter 1, '"The Stress of it All": Environment and People', Mary Kennedy explores work-related stress, which accounts for 37 per cent of work-related ill health and 45 per cent of days lost (Health and Safety Executive, HSE, 2016). Mary links the health and well-being of the practitioner with being an effective practitioner in the workplace. This link provides a rationale for urging the UK National Health Service to look after the staff in its employ. The chapter concludes by emphasising how tools such as mindfulness, Schwartz Rounds and Creative Learning Environments, when strategically embedded, can lead to improvements in organisational performance.

In Chapter 2, 'Embracing Change: A Continuing Process', Steve Wood looks at how we might embrace change, rather than be overwhelmed by it. Beginning with an examination of how change has been characterised in contemporary healthcare services, Steve offers several models that help to explain the change process. He then looks at some of the strategies that can help us survive the pummelling that healthcare staff receive from continuing change and innovation.

In Chapter 3, 'Nursing: A Profession with too Many Masters?', Peter J. Martin and Martin Harrison take a look at the political dimension of healthcare. 'The third person' in the room is the politician, who is 'virtually' present in every clinical encounter that we have with patients. The concept of an internalised and externalised locus of control (Rotter, 1954) is used to help think about what is and is not within our sphere of influence and control.

In Chapter 4, 'Reconnecting with Your Nursing Values', Cathy Constable helps us to revisit why we came into health and social care. This approach is used to help us measure the gap between our original aspirations and our current perception of our role. This chapter includes some exercises for those who find that they have recently lost their sense of direction.

In Chapter 5, 'Nursing and Mindfulness', Caroline Barratt and Tess Wagstaffe explore mindfulness as a practice for managing the stresses of the workplace. This chapter contains a number of practical exercises that support healthcare workers to develop greater awareness of their moment-to-moment experience and helps them notice when they are getting caught in habitual responses and mental chatter, enabling them to respond more creatively and to create moments of calm.

In Chapter 6, 'Thinking, Learning and Working under Fire', Steve Wood looks at the value of reflection and reflective practice as a reality check for our practice in maintaining a sense of a helicopter view of the practice environment. The chapter draws on some informal data collection from nurses about their experience and how they employ reflective techniques in everyday practice.

In Chapter 7, 'Self-Compassion', Tess Wagstaffe and Ness Woodcock-Dennis explore our self-perception and how, through an awareness of self-compassion, we can become kinder to ourselves. Health and social care workers deal with the emotional labour of practice, daily, and without this being managed effectively, people can quickly become overwhelmed by guilt and self-recrimination. The 'patient experience' is a cumulative process, involving many people and systems, but it is the person in face-to-face–patient contact who manages the fall-out when things are not perfect.

In Chapter 8, 'Collaborative Working', Mary Kennedy examines the complexity of delivering health and social care services. Many people will recognise stories of trying to work collaboratively, only to find that Information Systems do not 'speak' to each other or a different service paperwork meaning that detailed patient information must be transferred by hand. This chapter looks at barriers to collaboration and strategies for enhancing collaborative working.

In Chapter 9, 'Mental Parkour: Freeing the Mind', Martin Harrison and Peter J. Martin offer parkour (or free-running) as an analogy for how looking at the world from a different perspective enables health and social care practitioners to see matters differently. Such new perspectives can stimulate creativity and the generation of innovative approaches to problem-solving. The chapter also offers strategies to remain safe, whilst reconceptualising the world in which health and social care is delivered.

In Chapter 10, 'How your Past Influences your Present: The Unconscious at Work', Cathy Constable looks at how we might begin to manage the constant interaction between our conscious and unconscious worlds whilst in the workplace. The role of supervision and support networks are presented as strategies for managing this, often conflicted, process.

In the Chapter 11, 'Conclusion: Going Green – A Toolkit to Support Sustainable Practice', Peter J. Martin argues that individual interventions, however good, are ineffective if they are not part of a strategy to build sustainability into the individual and the workforce as a whole. All the themes and techniques outlined in the preceding chapters are presented in the form of a toolkit for building such sustainability. Bringing together these tools into an overarching strategy offers health and social care practitioners a way of thinking about practice and ultimately offers an aid to getting through the day without being harmed.

References

Health and Safety Executive (HSE) (2016) *Work-Related Stress, Anxiety and Depression: Statistics in Great Britain 2016*. London: HSE. Available at: http://qcompliance.co.uk/wp-content/uploads/2016/12/Work-related-Stress-Anxiety-and-Depression-Statistics-in-GB-2016.pdf (accessed July 2017).

Hochschild, A.R. (1983) *The Managed Heart: Commercialization of Human Feeling*. Berkeley and Los Angeles, CA: University of California Press.

Lave, J. and Wenger, E. (1991) *Situated Learning: Legitimate Peripheral Participation*. Cambridge: Cambridge University Press.

Nursing and Midwifery Council (NMC) (2010) *Standards for Pre-registration Nursing Education*. London: NMC.

NMC (2017) *Papers from Meetings – Council Meeting: 29 November 2017*. London: NMC.

Rotter, J.B. (1954) *Social Learning and Clinical Psychology*. New York: Prentice-Hall.

Schön, D. (1983) *The Reflective Practitioner*. San Francisco, CA: Jossey Bass.

1

'The Stress of It All'

Environment and People

Mary Kennedy

Nursing is a noble profession but too often a terrible job. (Chambliss, 1996: 1)

Chapter aims

- Explore the link between the health and well-being of nurses and the effect that this may have on the quality of patient care.
- Understand the benefits to the NHS of looking after the nurses' well-being.
- Appreciate what strategies could be employed by nurses to address work-related stress.

Introduction

Since Daniel F. Chambliss made the opening statement back in 1996, there have been significant changes in the delivery of healthcare and in nurse education. Therefore, could Chambliss's statement be considered a true reflection of nursing today?

There are few noble professions in the world but Chambliss considered nursing to be one of them. The *Oxford English Dictionary* (2017) defines noble as 'having or showing fine personal qualities or high moral principles', and there is no doubt that these are qualities that every nurse should possess. Those who choose nursing as a career enter a profession with substantial responsibility that involves dealing with people at vulnerable and significant moments in their lives. Nurses face many physical and emotional demands, and are often required to cope with difficult and challenging situations. To be able to efficiently and effectively deliver safe care, they must rely on their inherent qualities as well as on the ones that they acquire along the way in order to become what many consider to be the 'ideal' nurse.

So, why would such a 'noble' profession be considered a 'terrible job'? It has been proposed that nurses initially enter the profession with enthusiasm (Bjerknes and Bjørk, 2012), motivated by ideals and a sense of altruism (Maben, 2013). However, over time, these qualities can be eroded as nurses find themselves facing a variety of organisational difficulties, such as staff shortages, additional work demands, long hours and less supportive work environments (Bjerknes and Bjørk, 2012). When these factors are combined, not only do they hinder staff performance, as evidenced in recent NHS staff surveys (NHS, 2015a, 2015b), but they are also associated with high levels of work-related stress and burnout. Both stress and burnout are prevalent in nursing (Chana et al., 2015), and can lead to emotional exhaustion, depression, low job satisfaction and a decreased sense of personal effectiveness. Given such working conditions, it is understandable that some people may choose to agree with Chambliss and consider nursing to be 'a terrible job' (1996: 1).

Whatever view is taken, there are many nurses (including the author) who still take great satisfaction in their profession and consider it a privilege to be a nurse, caring for people at the most important moments of their lives. However, as a 'noble profession', should we allow the 'invasion' of stress and burnout to flourish within nursing? What are the consequences for the NHS if the well-being of nurses is neglected? As the NHS strives to provide high-quality, patient-centred care, it is vital that factors affecting nurses' health and well-being are investigated.

Stress in the NHS

Work-related stress is now a significant occupational health problem in the UK, accounting for 37 per cent of work-related ill health and 45 per cent of working days lost (Health and Safety Executive, HSE, 2016). According to the HSE (ibid.), stress, depression and anxiety, together represent the second most prevalent self-reported illness caused or made worse by work. An independent review into workplace mental health, commissioned by the UK government, explored how employers can better support all employees, including those with poor mental health or well-being, to remain in and thrive at work (Stevenson and Farmer, 2017). Key findings from the review highlighted that, although today there are more people at work with mental health conditions than ever before, 300,000 people with long-term mental health conditions lose their jobs each year (ibid.: 5). This is a much higher rate than those with physical health conditions. The review also estimated the cost of poor mental health to the UK economy at between £74 billion and £99 billion a year (ibid.: 5).

So, how does this relate to the NHS, the UK's largest employer, with more than 1.3 million employees. Suffice to say that all is not well and it's hardly surprising that the HSE (2016) have reported NHS staff as experiencing some of the highest levels of work-related stress. With increasing demands on services and growing financial pressures, the NHS is under enormous strain and there can be little doubt that such conditions have impacted on staffing levels, causing impossible workloads and subsequently affecting staff morale and levels of stress. Ultimately, demanding workloads and staff feeling overstretched and burnt out can erode compassion, affect quality of care, patient experience and patient outcomes (Care Quality Commission, CQC, 2017). Sadly, such findings are not new and the NHS has a history of being a stressful working environment (Boorman, 2009; NHS Staff Survey, 2015; 2016).

Reflective Question

What do you consider are the biggest challenges facing the NHS in the next five years?

Stress in the Workforce

Each year, the NHS completes a staff survey to collect information on how staff feel about their working environment. Over the last decade, the issue of health and well-being has been a key feature that has been discussed and scrutinised, but with apparently very little meaningful change. In 2009, the 'Boorman Review' (an independent review commissioned by the Department of Health, DH, see Boorman, 2009) explored the link between the health and well-being of NHS staff and the delivery of efficient and effective healthcare. At the time, the review found that 80 per cent of people working in the NHS in England felt that their health and well-being had an impact on patient care, but only 40 per cent felt that their employer was proactively trying to improve their health and well-being (ibid.: 35–36). The report also revealed that a quarter of NHS employees' absence from work was due to stress, anxiety and depression. A year later, findings from another NHS survey reported that staff felt that their physical health and emotional well-being affected their ability to undertake daily activities and their ability to care for patients.

Findings from the 2015 and 2016 NHS Staff Surveys were not dissimilar. In 2015, nearly 40 per cent of staff reported that, during the past twelve months, they had felt unwell because of work-related stress; 63 per cent reported that they had attended work in the previous three months despite not feeling well enough to perform their duties. Only 29 per cent felt that there were enough staff to enable them to conduct their role properly, with unplanned work steadily increasing; and 34 per cent said that their organisation took positive action on health and well-being (NHS Staff Survey, 2015: 6).

In 2016, the results on health and well-being were more encouraging, with 67 per cent of staff reporting that their manager took a positive interest in their individual health and well-being, and 90 per cent that their organisation 'definitely' or 'to some extent' took positive action. The proportion of staff who reported feeling unwell due to work-related stress was at its lowest reported level in five years but, nonetheless, was 37 per cent; and 60 per cent reported coming to work in the previous three months despite not feeling well enough to perform their duties or the requirements of their role. Although 92 per cent reported that this was a result of pressure from themselves rather than from other colleagues (20 per cent) or their manager (26 per cent), this figure is concerning in terms of safe practice and patient safety. The number of staff who reported working *unpaid* overtime each week was 59 per cent, which not only highlights the demands faced by NHS staff but also indicates their dedication to working above and beyond to keep the system going despite being under huge pressures (ibid., 2016: 4–5).

Key findings from the Royal College of Nursing (RCN) 2017 Employment Survey, based on the responses of 7720 members, would suggest that the unrelenting pressures faced by nurses on a daily basis continues to take its toll. For example, 'presenteeism' was found to be rising, with almost 48 per cent of those surveyed reporting that at least twice in the past year they had gone to work when feeling unwell; in 2013, the figure was 41 per cent; and 63 per cent of nurses said that they now face too much pressure at work compared to 53 per cent six years ago (RCN, 2017).

Reflective Question

What challenges your own clinical practice on a daily or regular basis?

It would appear obvious to suggest that the well-being of patients is dependent on the well being of the nurses providing their care. For nurses to provide compassionate care, they themselves must feel cared for, not only by each other but also by the organisation. This was a key finding from the Mid Staffordshire Inquiry (Francis, 2013), where senior leaders either ignored or weren't listening to the concerns of their own staff on issues around poor staffing and lack of resources. The inquiry brought a fresh focus on culture within NHS organisations, placing it at the heart of the fundamental care failings and addressing the need for a 'focus on culture of caring' (ibid.). Commenting at the time, Robert Francis (ibid.) emphasised the risks to patients when care becomes depersonalised and stressed the need for NHS organisations to be more open and transparent and willing to listen to both patients and staff:

> A common culture of serving and protecting patients and of rooting out poor practice will not spread throughout the system without insisting on openness, transparency and candour everywhere in it. (DH 2013d)

Reflective Question

What can be done to create caring cultures and supportive working environments?

In light of the Francis Report (ibid.), the need to understand what conditions influence and support nurses' caring behaviours is of vital importance. Addressing this, Chana et al. (2015) recommended the need to examine factors associated with nurses' levels of burnout, anxiety and depression, and quality of patient care, with the aim of providing suggestions to promote nursing staffs' well-being and enhance care-giving behaviours. This was echoed in a report from the Point of Care Foundation (PoCF, 2017), where the importance of NHS employers paying attention to staff and their experience at work was acknowledged. The message is clear: When staff feel positive and engaged it has a positive impact on patient experience.

Working in healthcare can be extremely rewarding, but it can also be emotionally and physically demanding, especially in the light of unprecedented and seemingly endless service pressures (Royal College of Physicians, 2015; PoCF, 2017). This can be linked to the critical shortage of nurses, a recurrent theme in recent years alongside issues of recruitment and retention. Data from a BBC Freedom of Information request revealed that between 2013 and 2015 in the NHS in England and Wales, there was a 50 per cent increase in nursing vacancies, up from 12,513 to 18,714. This trend has continued, and between 2016 and 2017, the Nursing and Midwifery (NMC) reported that for the first time, 45 per cent more UK registrants left the register than joined it. Such pressures have come at a time in today's healthcare when the complex and multifaceted needs of patients is particularly demanding (Ulrich et al., 2010). This is concerning because nursing, the largest proportion of the NHS workforce, with 585,404 nursing, midwifery and health visiting staff (NMC, 2017), is recognised as being one of the most stressful occupations (Lamont et al., 2017).

As pressures on the NHS continue to mount, ensuring the health and well-being of nurses is of increasing importance, especially if the NHS is to meet the many challenges that it faces. The financial implications are already clear, with the cost of staff absence due to poor health estimated at over £2.4 billion a year by Public Health England (PHE) (NHS England, 2017). This is before the additional cost of agency staff, or the cost of treatment, is taken into account (NHS England, 2015b). In an attempt to try and address the issues of staff health and well-being, NHS England's Chief Executive, Simon Stevens, launched a major initiative to try and support frontline staff and to improve workplace health (NHS England, 2015b).

Promoting Health and Well-Being in the Workplace

The World Health Organization (WHO) defines a healthy workplace as:

A healthy workplace is one in which workers and managers collaborate to use a continual improvement process to protect and promote the health, safety and well-being of all workers and the sustainability of the workplace by considering the following, based on identified needs:

- Health and safety concerns in the physical work environment;
- Health, safety and well-being concerns in the psychosocial work environment, including organisation of work and workplace culture;
- Personal health resources in the workplace; and
- Ways of participating in the community to improve the health of workers, their families and other members of the community. (WHO, 2010)

In order to help to achieve this aim, and to provide high-quality working environments, the NHS Constitution (DH, 2015) sets out a number of pledges (Table 1.1). One of the pledges is a commitment to: 'Provide support and opportunities for staff to maintain their health, well-being and safety.' Although many organisations have taken this commitment on board, there have been many others where staff are still reporting poor experiences, suggesting that the pledge has not become a reality for all and, so far, has been largely neglected (Maruthappu et al., 2015).

The stress of caring

In general, healthcare professionals are thought to have a high vulnerability to burn-out as a result of experiencing high levels of emotional strain owing to stressful

Table 1.1   The NHS Constitution for England (updated October 2015)

The NHS pledges to provide high-quality working environments for staff

1. To provide a positive working environment for staff and to promote supportive, open cultures that help staff do their job to the best of their ability

2. To provide all staff with clear roles and responsibilities and rewarding jobs for teams and individuals that make a difference to patients, their families and carers and communities

3. To provide all staff with personal development, access to appropriate education and training for their jobs, and line management support to enable them to fulfil their potential

4. To provide support and opportunities for staff to maintain their health, wellbeing and safety

5. To engage staff in decisions that affect them and the services they provide, individually, through representative organisations and through local partnership working arrangements. All staff will be empowered to put forward ways to deliver better and safer services for patients and their families (pledge)

6. To have a process for staff to raise an internal grievance (pledge)

7. To encourage and support all staff in raising concerns at the earliest reasonable opportunity about safety, malpractice or wrongdoing at work, responding to and, where necessary, investigating the concerns raised and acting consistently with the Employment Rights Act 1996

working environments. However, compared to other health-care professionals, nurses are found to experience higher levels of burnout and psychological distress, which is thought to be closely linked to their caring behaviours (Chana et al., 2015). Burnout is usually thought of as an individual's response to prolonged work-related stress, which, in turn, impacts on job satisfaction and, thereafter, can often affect productivity, performance, turnover and well-being among healthcare professionals and other kinds of workers (Stevenson and Farmer, 2017). In nursing, owing to the nature of the work, this can be attributed to prolonged direct personal contact of an emotional nature, such as illness, suffering and death. The PoCF (2017) have expressed the view that if staff are placed under sustained pressure and feel unable to offer patients the care that they need, then they can suffer so-called 'moral distress' and their sensitivity to stress and burnout is heightened. When staff find themselves working in very demanding environments with little control or support, 'toxic environments' can develop as staff struggle to cope (ibid.). Such arguments are not new and were identified in the late 1970s by the sociologist Robert Karasek (1979, cited in Van der Doef and Maes, 1999), who conceived the concept of the 'Job Demand Control Model' (Figure 1.1). This showed that job strain occurs in work environments that have a lot of demands, coupled with little control. Karasek's model defined high-stress, unhealthy jobs as those with low control and high demand conditions, reflective of the positions that many nurses find themselves in on a daily basis.

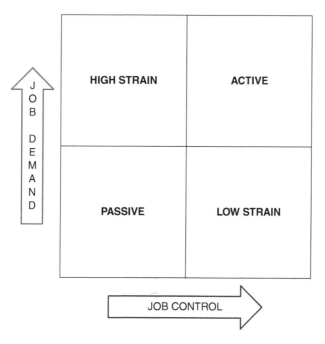

Figure 1.1 Job Demand Control Model (adapted from Karasek, 1979, cited in Van der Doef and Maes, 1999)

There is increasing recognition that all staff are affected by the emotional demands of caring for patients, whether they are frontline clinical staff, associated healthcare professionals or non-clinicians (PoCF, 2017), and that rates of work-related anxiety and depression continue to rise (Stevenson and Farmer, 2017). Back in 2008, the Department of Health commissioned a major piece of research in order to understand what mattered to staff in the NHS by exploring the factors, especially emotional ones, that drive advocacy, motivation and the delivery of excellent services. Findings from the research identified that staff commitment, engagement and productivity were linked to four main themes:

- The resources to deliver quality care.
- The support needed to do a good job.
- A worthwhile job that offers the chance to develop.
- The opportunity to improve team-working.

In the review by Stevenson and Farmer (2017) into mental health in the workplace, a series of recommendations were made, setting out core principles and standards that all employers should commit to if mentally healthy work environments are to become a reality (Table 1.2). Paul Farmer, the Chief Executive of Mind and one of the report's reviewers, said:

> The human cost of failing to address mental health in the workplace is clear. Workplace mental health should be a priority for organisations across the UK. Every employer in the UK has a responsibility to support employees with mental health problems and promote the mental well-being of their entire workforce. (Mind, 2017)

The NHS, which employs over 1.3 million staff, has a key role and responsibility to lead the way in driving this forward alongside other national agendas, such as the initiative proposed by Simon Steven's NHS England's Chief Executive (2015b) for healthy workplace environments.

Table 1.2   Thriving at Work: Mental Health Core Standards

1. Produce, implement and communicate a mental health at work plan

2. Develop mental health awareness among employees

3. Encourage open conversations about mental health and the support available when employees are struggling

4. Provide employees with good working conditions and ensure they have a healthy work–life balance and opportunities for development

5. Promote effective people management through line managers and supervisors

6. Routinely monitor employee mental health and wellbeing

The emotional labour of care

Professional caring involves emotional labour, which Hochschild defined as: 'the induction or suppression of a feeling in order to produce in other people a sense of being cared for in a safe place' (cited in Smith, 2012: 11). This kind of labour can be overwhelming and nurses can become stressed and less able to induce or suppress their feelings, and may instead avoid situations that require this behaviour. The notion that nursing staff dehumanise and distance themselves from those under their care is not new and was introduced by the psychoanalyst Isabel Menzies in 1960 (cited in Smith, 2012: 11). In her research into why students were leaving nursing, Menzies identified high levels of anxiety as being partly responsible. Through her research, she demonstrated how nurses organised their work to reduce emotional labour by splitting contact with patients into tasks in a way that is often seen as the antithesis of compassionate care (Smith, 2012). Commenting on this definitive piece of nursing literature, Lawlor (2009) summarised the defensive techniques that Menzies identified (Table 1.3).

In reviewing the research paper by Menzies, Lawlor (2009) questions whether it passes the 'test of time' and believed that, yes, it did. Interestingly, even though Lawlor's (ibid.) own work was published nearly a decade ago, his own views are still as relevant in today's healthcare as they were when Menzies conducted her research in the 1960s. In a similar picture to today's, she reported high levels of stress in the system and high sickness rates:

> the direct impact on the nurse of physical illness is intensified by her task of meeting and dealing with psychological distress in other people, including her own colleagues. It is by no means easy to tolerate such stress even if one is not under similar stress oneself ... (Menzies, 1960, cited in Lawlor, 2009: 524)

Table 1.3   Menzies' Social Defence Systems (adapted from Lawlor, 2009)

1. Splitting up the nurse–patient relationship
2. Depersonalisation, categorisation and denial of the significance of the individual
3. Detachment and denial of feelings
4. The attempt to eliminate decisions by ritual task-performance
5. Reducing the weight of responsibility in decision-making by checks and counterchecks
6. Collusive social redistribution of responsibility and irresponsibility
7. Purposeful obscurity in the formal distribution of responsibility
8. The reduction of the impact of responsibility by delegation to superiors
9. Idealisation and underestimation of personal development possibilities
10. Avoidance of change

Beating the stress invasion

The evidence shows that the well-being of patients is highly dependent on the well-being of staff (Chana et al., 2015) but for staff to provide care with compassion, they themselves must feel cared for and supported in their work (Goodrich, 2012). Effective staff support and management are vital to creating a positive and engaging culture, as they are directly related to patient experience and quality of care (Dixon-Woods et al., 2014). Clearly, senior leaders have a key role in facilitating supportive, caring cultures (Rafferty et al., 2015).

Following the public enquiries into a number of failing NHS Trusts, including those carried out by Keogh (2013), Francis (2013) and Berwick (2013), there has been a much stronger emphasis in the NHS on valuing and engaging with staff in order to support safe, effective, compassionate care. Specifically, within nursing, the model of the 6Cs has been developed to encourage 'Compassion in Practice' (Cummings and Bennett, 2012). These are:

- Care
- Compassion
- Courage
- Communication
- Commitment
- Competence

In order to support the creation of healthy working environments, there are a number of initiatives that staff can adopt, either individually, as part of a team or within peer support.

Mindfulness

In recent years, the practice of mindfulness has been the subject of increased attention and interest due to the growing evidence base demonstrating that it can be an effective method for treating many mental and physical health conditions, as well as generally improving well-being (Mental Health Foundation, 2010). 'Mindfulness' has been defined by Kabat-Zinn as, 'a way of paying attention in the present moment, intentionally and non-judgmentally' (1994: 4), and has its origins in Buddhist tradition. Within healthcare, the potential of mindfulness to help reduce burnout or fatigue has been recognised and is discussed in more detail in Chapter 5 (Barratt and Wagstaffe). Reviewing the benefits of mindfulness, the authors suggest that healthcare professionals should be encouraged to develop their practice of mindfulness as this can be beneficial in relieving stress and increasing attention levels and awareness. Although they recommend several activities that you can attempt, you may also find the 'ABCs of mindfulness' a useful tool to complement these (Table 1.4).

Table 1.4 The ABCs of mindfulness: A tool for daily use

A is for awareness. Becoming more aware of what you are thinking and doing – what is going on in your mind and body.

B is for just 'being' with your experience. Avoiding the tendency to respond on auto-pilot and feed problems by creating your own story.

C is for 'seeing' things and responding more wisely. By creating a gap between the experience and our reaction we can make wiser choices.

Source: Juliet Adams, founder of Mindfulnet. Available at: www.mindfulnet.org/page2.htm

Schwartz Rounds

(**Schwartz Rounds**® Reproduced with permission.)

Another approach to tackling the emotional burden of healthcare is to introduce Schwartz Rounds, which provide staff with a safe and facilitated space to discuss the emotional and social aspects of working in healthcare. Created by the Schwartz Center for Compassionate Healthcare® in Boston, MA, Schwartz Rounds are recognised as an evidence-based initiative to improve patient experience. They were recognised by the Department of Health (2013e) and the Francis Report (2013) as a mechanism for improving team-building and cohesiveness. In the UK, Schwartz Rounds are supported by the Point of Care Foundation under license from the USA-based Schwartz Center and work with over 200 organisations across the UK and Ireland (PoCF, 2017).

The PoCF recommend Schwartz Rounds as a compassionate collaborative practice and an education model that can be used to innovate team relationships, stimulate learning and improve care outcomes. During Schwartz Rounds, staff are provided with the opportunity to openly and honestly discuss the psychological, emotional and social issues that they face in caring for patients and their families – the human dimension of healthcare. Schwartz Rounds are not about seeking solutions, but are about reflection and enabling staff to feel more connected to their colleagues and their own values and commitment to caring.

Creating Learning Environments for Compassionate Care (CLECC)

Designed to promote compassionate care, Creating Learning Environments for Compassionate Care (CLECC) is a model that is a ward-based practice development programme. The focus is on developing sustainable ward management and team practices that enhance the capacity to provide compassionate care, emphasising the importance of staff well-being in the provision of high-quality care (Bridges and Fuller, 2015).

Conclusion

The Department of Health and NHS England are committed to being a model employer and to creating healthy workplace environments (DH, 2015; NHS England, 2015b). However, it important not to forget that this is a road well trodden and at times there is sense of dejà vu. This is captured in Lawlor's (2009: 530) closing remarks when he reflected on the impact of Menzies' classic paper on nursing and wrote the following:

> But the paper seems to have had less of an impact on policy makers and those responsible for designing organisational systems for health and social care. The emphasis on targets, and the increase in volume of work in all of our health and social care systems, do not seem to take into account the psychological impact of such changes on the organisational system and the staff who work in it. For instance, the obsession of senior staff with reaching targets, rather than with the quality of care, has led in certain hospitals in the UK recently to a demoralised staff group and the death of patients. This illustrates the kind of split between senior policy makers and practitioners on the ground which Menzies warned us about 50 years ago.

Let's hope that, in the next 50 years, nurses are no longer reporting similar experiences and that high levels of stress and burnout are things of the past. Achieving this ambition is important for the health and well-being of all staff and of the quality of care delivered.

References

Berwick, D. (2013). *A Promise to Learn: A Commitment to Act: Improving the Safety of Patients in England*. London: Department of Health.

Bjerknes, M.S. and Bjørk, I.T. (2012) 'Entry into nursing: An ethnographic study of newly qualified nurses taking on the nursing role in a hospital setting', *Nursing Research and Practice*, 2012, Article ID 690348.

Boorman, S. (2009) *NHS and Well-Being: Final Report, November 2009*. London: Stationery Office.

Bridges, J. and Fuller, A. (2015) 'Creating learning environments for compassionate care: A programme to promote compassionate care by health and social care teams', *International Journal of Older People Nursing*, 10: 48–58.

Care Quality Commission (CQC) (2017) *The State of Health Care and Adult Social Care in England, 2016/17*. London: CQC. Available at: www.gov.uk/government/publications (accessed August 2017).

Chambliss, D.F. (1996) *Beyond Caring: Hospitals, Nurses, and the Social Organization of Ethics*. Chicago, IL: University of Chicago Press.

Chana, N., Kennedy, P. and Chessell, Z.J. (2015) 'Nursing staffs' emotional well-being and caring behaviours', *Journal of Clinical Nursing*, 24: 2835–48.

Cummings, J. and Bennett, V. (2012) *Compassion in Practice, Nursing, Midwifery and Care Staff: Our Vision and Strategy*. London: Department of Health.

Department of Health (DH) (2008) *What Matters to Staff in the NHS*. London: DH. Available at: http://webarchive.nationalarchives.gov.uk/20130124043049/www.dh.gov.uk/prod_consum_dh/groups/dh_digitalassets/@dh/@en/documents/digitalasset/dh_085535.pdf (accessed September 2017).

DH (2013d) *Mid Staffordshire NHS Foundation Trust Public Inquiry: Openness and Transparency*. London: DH. Available at: https://engage.dh.gov.uk/francisresponse/openness-and-transparency/ (accessed 12 March 2018).

DH (2013e) *Expansion of groundbreaking scheme to support NHS staff*. Press release. Available at: www.gov.uk/government/news/expansion-of-groundbreaking-scheme-to-support-nhs-staff (accessed 12 March 2018).

DH (2015) *The NHS Constitution for England*. London: DH. Available at: www.gov.uk/government/publications/the-nhs-constitution-for-england/the-nhs-constitution-for-england (accessed July 2017).

Dixon-Woods, M., Baker, R., Charles, K. et al. (2014) 'Culture and behaviour in the English National Health Service: Overview of lessons from a large multimethod study', *BMJ Quality & Safety*, 23: 106–15. Available at: http://dx.doi.org/10.1136/bmjqs-2013-002471 (accessed August 2017).

Francis, R. (2013) *Report of the Mid Staffordshire NHS Foundation Trust Public Inquiry, Vol. 1: Analysis of Evidence and Lessons Learned (Part 1)*, HC 898-I. London: The Stationery Office. Available at: http://webarchive.nationalarchives.gov.uk/20150407084003/www.midstaffspublicinquiry.com/sites/default/files/report/Volume%201.pdf (accessed 10 March 2017).

Goodrich, J. (2012) 'Supporting hospital staff to provide compassionate care: do Schwartz Center Rounds work in English hospitals?', *Journal of the Royal Society of Medicine*, 105: 117–122.

Health and Safety Executive (HSE) (2016) *Work Related Stress, Anxiety and Depression Statistics in Great Britain 2016*. Available at: http://qcompliance.co.uk/wp-content/uploads/2016/12/Work-related-Stress-Anxiety-and-Depression-Statistics-in-GB-2016.pdf (accessed 24 April 2018).

Kabat-Zinn, J. (1994) *Wherever You Go, There You Are: Mindfulness Meditation for Everyday Life*. New York: Hyperion.

Keogh, B. (2013) *Review into the Quality of Care and Treatment Provided by 14 Hospital Trusts in England: overview report*. London: NHS.

Lamont, S. et al. (2017) '"Mental health day" sickness absence amongst nurses and midwives: Workplace, workforce, psychosocial and health characteristics', *Journal of Advanced Nursing*, 73: 1172–81.

Lawlor, D. (2009) 'Test of time, a case study in the functioning of social systems as a defence against anxiety: Rereading 50 years on', *Clinical Child Psychology and Psychiatry*, 14: 523–9.

Maben, J. (2013) 'Staff must be supported to put patient care first', Comment, *Health Service Journal*. Available at: www.hsj.co.uk/comment/staff-must-be-supported-to-put-patient-care-first/5064105.article (accessed July 2017).

Maruthappu, M., Sood, H. and Black, C. (2015) 'Prioritising prevention and the health of NHS staff', *The Lancet*, 386: 1322–32.

Mental Health Foundation (2010) *Be Mindful Report*. London: Mental Health Foundation.

Mind (2017) *Stevenson-Farmer Independent Review into Workplace Mental Published*. Available at: https://www.mind.org.uk/news-campaigns/news/stevenson-farmer-independent-review-into-workplace-mental-health-published/#.WqZSheRLGUl (accessed 12 March 2018).

NHS England (2015a) *NHS Staff Health & Wellbeing: CQUIN 2017–19 Indicator 1 Implementation Support*. London: NHS England. Available at: www.england.nhs.uk/wp-content/uploads/2017/10/staff-health-wellbeing-cquin-2017-19-implementation-support.pdf (accessed September 2017).

NHS England (2015b) 'Simon Stevens announces major drive to improve health in NHS workplace', News, 2 September. Available at: www.england.nhs.uk/2015/09/02/nhs-workplace (accessed September 2017).

NHS England (2017) *NHS staff health & wellbeing: CQUIN 2017-19 Indicator 1 Implementation Support*. Available at: www.england.nhs.uk/wp-content/uploads/2017/10/staff-health-wellbeing-cquin-2017-19-implementation-support.pdf (accessed 12 March 2018).

NHS Staff Survey (2015) Available at: www.nhsstaffsurveys.com/Page/1021/Past-Results/Historical-Staff-Survey-Results/ (accessed September 2017).

NHS Staff Survey (2016) Available at: www.nhsstaffsurveys.com/Page/1006/Latest-Results/2016-Results/ (accessed September 2017).

Nursing and Midwifery Council (NMC) (2017) 'New figures show an increase in numbers of nurses and midwives leaving the professions', 3 July. Available at: www.nmc.org.uk/news/news-and-updates/new-figures-show-an-increase-in-numbers-of-nurses-and-midwives-leaving-the-professions/ (accessed September 2017).

Oxford English Dictionary (OED) (2017) Oxford: Oxford University Press.

Point of Care Foundation (PoCF) (2017) *Behind Closed Doors: Can We Expect NHS Staff to Be the Shock Absorbers of a System under Pressure?* London: Point of Care Foundation. Available at: https://16682-presscdn-0-1-pagely.netdna-ssl.com/wp-content/uploads/2017/07/POC_Closed_doors_07_17_v5.pdf (December 2017).

Rafferty, A.M., Xyrichis, A. and Caldwell, C. (2015) *Post-graduate Education and Career Pathways in Nursing: A Policy Brief*. London: King's College London.

Royal College of Nursing (RCN) (2017) 'The domino effect: The RCN reveals the results of its latest employment survey', RCN Bulletin, 29 November. Available at: www.rcn.org.uk/magazines/bulletin/2017/december/employment-survey (accessed December 2017).

Royal College of Physicians (2015) *Work and Wellbeing in the NHS: Why Staff Health Matters to Patient Care*. London: Royal College of Physicians. Available at: file:///C:/Users/jgrogan/Downloads/Work%20and%20wellbeing%20in%20the%20NHS.PDF (accessed October 2017).

Smith, P. (2012) *The Emotional Labour of Nursing Revisited: Can Nurses Still Care?* London: Palgrave Macmillan.

Stevenson, R. and Farmer, P. (2017) *Thriving at Work: The Stevenson/Farmer Review of Mental Health and Employers*. London: Department for Work and Pensions (DWP) and (DH). Available at: www.gov.uk/government/uploads/system/uploads/attachment_data/file/658145/thriving-at-work-stevenson-farmer-review.pdf (accessed October 2017).

Ulrich, C.M, Taylor, C., Soeken, K. et al. (2010) 'Everyday ethics: Ethical issues and stress in nursing practice', *Journal of Advanced Nursing*, 66: 2510–19.

van der Doef, M. and Maes, S. (1999) 'The Job Demand-Control (-Support) Model and psychological well-being: A review of 20 years of empirical research', *Work & Stress*, 13(2): 87–114.

World Health Organization (WHO) (2010) *Healthy Workplaces: A Model for Action for Employers – For Employers, Workers, Policy-Makers and Practitioners*. Geneva: WHO. Available at: www.who.int/occupational_health/publications/healthy_workplaces_model_action.pdf (accessed November 2017).

2

Embracing Change

A Continuing Process

Steve Wood

Change is the only constant in life. (Heraclitus)

Chapter aims

- Describe the context of change in contemporary healthcare.
- Explain how change is the result of social, political, professional and demographic factors outside of the individual's control.
- Outline how change and the rate of change can affect the individual.
- Explain how nurses can employ positive strategies in order to cope with change in clinical practice.

Introduction

The current level of public and media scrutiny and the rate of change in the care sector are unprecedented, and this can adversely affect the individual nurse. Such an impact results from a combination of social, political, professional and demographic factors outside of the nurse's control but, nonetheless, the effects of these changes have to be responded to. The impact of this on the nurse is explored in the context of theories of stress reactions and change frameworks and Brandon's (1991) explanation of 'innovation without change'. Is 'refreezing', as espoused by Kurt Lewin (Lewin and Gold, 1999), still possible in contemporary healthcare or is constant movement the new refreezing? In which case, should coping with movement now be the focus for change management? If so, what might help nurses deal with constant change? Positive strategies can be used to deal with, and influence, change in contemporary clinical practice and some of these are outlined. Nursing has a strong collective voice, and this can also be used to influence the culture of health-care organisations.

The Context of Change in Contemporary Healthcare

> What a high personal price some of them are paying for doing this job, in this context, right now. (Wren 2016: 87)

The pace of change in contemporary healthcare is undoubtedly stressful and can often feel overwhelming for nurses working at the clinical interface. This may give an impression of trying to operate in a 'perfect storm' of competing factors such as the expectation to use new technological innovations, cope with resource shortages, respond to quality inspections and Trust mergers, meet clinical targets, complete care documentation and address patient expectations while being concurrently expected to provide high-quality, person-centred care.

It is worthwhile considering some of the fundamental driving forces for this 'perfect storm' scenario and to assess the potential impact on practice. The reader is probably acutely aware of many of these, but it can be useful to take a reflective perspective so as to help reframe the stressors and to explore potential new ways of responding to these. To compound this situation, a perusal through the United Kingdom Department of Health website reveals more than seventeen current policies, with a high number of these being either reviewed or released in the last five years. Additionally, a search of a typical NHS Trust website showed that staff must incorporate around seventy-five clinical policies into their practice.

Such clinical policies are designed to reflect the fact that the health status of the UK population is changing, and it is becoming more challenging for health and social care providers to meet the needs fully of service users. This situation has been caused mainly by an ageing population and an increase in the number of people living longer (Office for National Statistics, 2017). This means that the NHS is expected to treat more people than ever before, with the numbers projected to accelerate.

These factors should be considered, first in the context of 20 per cent of nurses choosing not to renew their registration since the Nursing and Midwifery Council (NMC) introduced revalidation in April 2016. Second, with a reduction of 96 per cent of European Union nurses registering to work in the UK following the announcement of the UK's separation from the European Union ('Brexit'). Consequently, it is little wonder that the pressure on nurses has significantly increased.

Further to this, the NMC introduced a new version of The Code in March 2015, which regulates nursing practice. Additional NMC clinical guidelines that nurses must incorporate into their role have been produced, and standards for education and practice learning have also been reviewed.

All these NMC initiatives have impacted on nurses and, in the case of revalidation, have potentially required nurses to take time away from clinical practice. Whilst continuing professional development and reflective practice are an essential part of maintaining skilful and knowledgeable practice, on the whole, no additional time or study resources is allocated for this purpose. Indeed, the opposite seems to have occurred, with cuts to education budgets for study opportunities.

Similarly, the 2017 cyberattack on the NHS demonstrated not only its over-reliance on, and poor management of, information technology (IT) but also the importance of finding new ways of utilising IT. Recent developments, such as the use of tablet computers to document care events remotely and the use of technological advancements in respect of new equipment for inpatient care, all exemplify how nurses are required to adapt and develop new skills. Such expectations coexist with acute pressures in clinical practice, including staff shortages, the implementation of new roles such as nurse associates and apprenticeship schemes, different mentorship requirements such as coaching and new ways of operating shift patterns.

How change harms us: The personal impact of change

The above are no more than examples of current pressures and are not intended to be a comprehensive list because, most likely, these only represent the tip of the ice-berg. I am sure that you are adding many more examples as you read this. However, the outcome of this scenario is that clinicians are under an ever-increasing burden of expectation. Nurses often express their experiences of change in contemporary healthcare practice in blogs and social media. Such experiences describe feeling drained of compassion and being undervalued and under stress.

The response of NHS leaders to these perspectives and increasing awareness of the pressure of working in healthcare services seems to have been a call for the development of higher resilience on the part of care workers. 'Resilience' appears to have become the latest buzzword and, in consequence, it seems to have become accepted that the development of greater resilience will provide the solution rather than examining the organisational and political origins of the problem. This then focuses the issue on the individual rather than the system that perpetuates it. For now, let's put aside the concept of resilience and instead re-examine the impact of the many current changes on the individual nurse in the context of some traditional psychological explanations.

The Holmes and Rahe Stress Scale, also known as the Social Readjustment Rating Scale (SRRS), is concerned with evaluating the long-term effects of prolonged stress (Hockenbury and Hockenbury, 2006). It is suggested that the central tenets of this tool still have significant relevance. This scale gives a rating, or score, to all the stressors currently occurring in a person's life, including personal, social and work factors. Each stressor on its own might seem relatively minor, but if several occur at the same time, then there is the potential for overload and acute distress. Each person will respond differently but if a significant life event occurs at the same time as other life events, then the person will most likely experience excessive stress and so will feel overloaded. Such situations can commonly arise in a typical working week for nurses or even during just one shift.

Similarly, the Yerkes-Dodson Law describes how, if there is a lack of external stimulation, then we become lethargic and bored (Chaskalson, 2011). Therefore, I am sorry to say that a level of stress or change is essential for performance! However, if we are overstressed or overloaded, then after a certain point, our standard of performance in practice will decline (ibid.).

You often hear nurses express their displeasure at having to deal with the multiple external pressures of clinical work by indicating that their primary task is just to provide a high quality of care. Such sentiments and the inherent pressures and stressors all contribute to what Festinger (1962) called 'cognitive dissonance'. This phenomenon is concerned with incidents that question our belief systems and attitudes. In such circumstances, the only way in which this psychological discomfort can be resolved is by adjusting our outlook and thereby regaining control. As outlined and explained by George Kelly (2013 [1959]) in his Personal Construct theory, we develop our own unique constructs or values from experience and then utilise these to interpret and control new events. When situations are challenging, we then use our constructs to regain control (Carver and Scheier, 2012). Consider this concept in the context of the new Sustainability and Transformation Partnerships (STPs), which are 44 partnerships between the NHS and local councils in England and have been formed to improve healthcare based not only on the requirements of care providers but also on the local population's needs. These could be viewed as an attempt to reduce spending on the NHS or, alternatively, as a platform to create innovative thinking about the way in which the NHS should be managed and resourced for future generations. Either way, the STPs have challenged our thinking about care, and so the dissonance must be resolved.

As can be seen from the stress reaction theories above, it is quite reasonable to feel the impact of these pressures personally, and it is entirely understandable that nurses may feel stressed and overwhelmed at work. Overload resulting from multiple stressors will cause this. Explanations for how such reactions can be more efficiently dealt with in current healthcare can be seen in both established and 'new' change management theories and models. For example, Lippitt et al. (1958) sees the change process moving through seven phases but considers the role of the 'change agent' to be central to diagnosing the problem, assessing the motivation for change, defining the stages, ensuring that there is role clarity for all participants and implementing gradual change in order to ensure that it becomes integral to organisational culture. Similarly, Rogers (1995) identifies five phases of change, namely awareness, interest, evaluation, trial and adoption.

Lewin's seminal work on change, the 'Three-Step Change Theory' (Lewin and Gold, 1999), emerged in the late 1940s. However, his framework continues to be taught in change management courses and is still frequently utilised to help plan, implement and evaluate change in healthcare. Lewin and Gold (1999) describe the process of moving from the individual's initial reluctance to change by 'unfreezing' their resistance. To do this, force field analysis is utilised, whereby motivating and resisting forces are assessed. The motivating forces are then worked on and resisting forces reduced by the change agent(s) so as to facilitate 'movement' of the person's behaviour and attitudes. Once the desired change has been attained, then the focus is on using 'refreezing' strategies so as to ensure the change pervades.

Lewin's ideas remain credible and widely used, but if these are applied to contemporary clinical practice, it becomes questionable if 'refreezing' can still be achieved. While this change framework might again help explain why nurses experience dissonance and stress, it is possible that constant 'movement' or change or even chaos has now become the new constant. It is interesting to reflect on this observation in respect of its similarity to Discordianism, a movement that was established in the late 1950s and that sees the Greek goddess of discord, Eris, as a mythological symbol. Discordianism asserts that rather than stability, in fact, the only consistent state is chaos, change, confusion and uncertainty. Therefore, it is chaos or change that should be embraced as an important part of our experience and reality (Higgs, 2012). In which case, perhaps, coping with 'movement' should be the focus for change management rather than attempting to achieve a stable state. The importance of responding in a more dynamic way to change on both a personal and operational level was highlighted by Welch, who stated that:

> We've long believed that when the rate of change inside an institution becomes slower than the rate of change outside, the end is in sight. The only question is when. (2000: 4)

If change and being exposed to prolonged levels of stress correlates with contemporary healthcare work, then the next consideration should be how such stress and change may harm us as individuals and as nurses. The 'change curve', based on Kubler-Ross's (1969) model, which explains the grieving process, has also been correlated with the change process and stress reactions. There are now several versions of the change curve, but all move through the original stages of the grief reaction, namely shock and denial, anger and depression, acceptance and integration. Following this final stage, there is a sense of optimism and of progress being made. It has been suggested that a self-assessment of the stage in which you are at and where others are in the change curve could be useful. However, the limitations of this framework seem to be the same as Lewin's framework, in that it presupposes that following a change, there is a period of stability. The need to conduct a self-assessment of where you are in the change process also seems apparent in the work of Rogers (1995), who asks individuals to self-appraise their likelihood to become involved in change and the roles they might play (Table 2.1).

How did you do? Were you an innovator or a laggard? Perhaps these descriptions need to be updated!

Burnout and Emotional Labour

Other well-known and extensively researched effects of prolonged stress in nursing are concerned with the phenomena of burnout and the emotional labour of care work. These are essential influencing factors and, again, as these have been widely documented, there is no intention to review the literature here, other than to briefly summarise and reflect on the reasons why these occur and how nurses who are experiencing these might be supported and helped.

Table 2.1 Roles in the change process (Rogers, 1995)

Ideal Type	Per cent	Description of Ideal Type
Innovators	10	Champions who are prepared to take a risk, and see what happens
Early adopters	15	Follow innovators or because they see the benefits of change
Early majority	25	Not particularly vocal, but are likely to commit with solid evidence
Late majority	25	Cautious, wait-and-see attitude before they are ready to commit
Laggards or resistors	25	Resist or challenge because they have a strong stake in the outcome. If they can be convinced that the change is necessary and valuable it will succeed, can influence others

Burnout in nursing has been defined by Maslach as: 'a multi-dimensional construct comprised of emotional exhaustion, depersonalisation and diminished personal competence that occurs among those who do "people work" of some kind' (1982: 3). Suggested causes of this include the continuing stressful nature of the work and having to cope with the emotional aspects of nursing such as end-of-life care and helping people adjust to a long-term illness, working in a culture of care that is unsupportive and one that does not facilitate openness about the difficulties faced, pressurised care environments and corresponding increased workloads, shift and work patterns and the implications of nursing as a calling, which results in neglecting to care for oneself (Khamisa et al., 2015). The high levels of stress and levels of burnout seen in nursing have also been correlated with the consequences of the 'emotional labour of nursing', whereby powerful emotions that result from caring situations go unresolved owing to a lack of sufficient support systems (Sawbridge and Hewison, 2011). Burnout can affect even the most committed and dedicated nurses and is also high among newly qualified nurses (Health Education England, 2014). Travaglia et al. (2011) further describe how change fatigue results from mergers, restructuring and a lack of equity in organisational cultures and that then produce barriers to change.

Therefore, it can be seen that the potential long-term emotional implications of prolonged stress and excessive change for nurses are clear and this results in 'change weariness'. Perhaps, then, it is possible to think differently about the nature of some nursing or care interventions and the 'energy' expended on these. There seems to be a consensus that the focus for nursing should be on delivering person-centred care that is reflective of what service users want from providers. Both are a requirement of all current health and social care policies and the numerous patient and family carer surveys, declarations and bills of rights that outline exactly what people want from services.

Consider these in the context of Brandon's (1991) 'match or mismatch'. Brandon undertook a survey of professionals, asking what they thought service users wanted from mental health providers. At the same time, he asked care recipients what they wanted from services. When Brandon compared the two lists, there was no match or any similarity in the expressed needs, hence 'match or mismatch'. The clinicians suggested that service users wanted increased access to treatment, medication and inpatient care, whereas care recipients wanted improved community and social support. Contemporary examples of Brandon's observations within dementia care could include the proliferation of carer education (itself an oxymoron) or support groups that require relatives to attend a centre, when their primary preferred need is more efficient post-diagnostic support and continuing contact.

In a more significant way, there is now widespread agreement on what person-centred care should consist of and that this should be a central component of high-quality, individualised nursing care. The values and principles proposed by Kitwood (1997) still underpin contemporary person-centred care frameworks, and the work of Brooker (2007) has further updated Kitwood's ideas by emphasising the importance of the care environment and culture. However, despite this agreement, it seems that care practices are frequently presented by nurses as 'person-centred' but, on closer scrutiny, these do not appear either to conform to or to comply with current definitions of person-centred care that require the full involvement of patients at all stages, namely in the design, planning, implementation and evaluation of any intervention.

Therefore, person-centred care principles are aspired to by care services and nurses but rarely achieved. Possible causes of this include organisational and management structures, commissioning pressures and team-working barriers that prevent services from complying with contemporary person-centred principles and delivering what people with service users ask for from care providers. Such a phenomenon is similar to another concept put forward by Brandon, namely 'innovation without change', whereby 'being busy' is translated into the mistaken belief that 'innovative' practice is taking place because of the high levels of activity. Bear in mind that service users would often not choose the services being offered, and so care is organised for the benefit of clinicians rather than patients under the pretext of being person-centred. The outcome of these types of activities is that considerable time and effort is being expended that does not meet the needs of care recipients. An example of this was evident in the 2017 Sepsis Awareness Week, which showed improvements in the hospital screening and assessment but no corresponding advances in treatment and interventions or reduction in incidence.

Reflective Question

Think about your own clinical team and try to identify if similar activities are being utilised that purport to be innovative but only result in the opposite being achieved?

How we survive change

Helping nurses cope with change would undoubtedly reduce anxiety and reinforce the idea that it takes more effort to fight change than to accept it. It is also possible that, on occasion, the benefits of change may not be apparent. An example of this might be the current move to a paperless care documentation system. Many practical difficulties are often cited about such a move, but a positive outcome of this strategy could be broader and easier access to patient records.

Several contemporary theorists writing about implementing change in healthcare services tend to focus on identifying barriers to change, how to overcome resistance and how to manage staff who are unwilling to change (de Silva, 2015). However, such a stance has the potential to undermine the professional integrity and autonomy of nurses, and so more creative and innovative approaches are needed to cope with constant change. Indeed, creative thinking is now considered integral to balancing the need for change and opportunity, with consideration of both organisational risk and personal impact.

The concept of 'creative change' is the enabling of creative thinking within organisations, as proposed by (Mueller, 2017). Such a strategy is based on how successful organisations acknowledge the difficulties in executing the creative concepts put forward by their staff through establishing structures that facilitate the implementation of these ideas (ibid.). This type of creative strategy is useful because it can simultaneously achieve cultural change by enabling the involvement of participants and the fostering of partnership. These innovative approaches also support the notion that change does not have to be a negative experience and that there are many practice benefits of change, including improved communication patterns and teamwork, enhanced patient care and reduced staff turnover and sickness rates (Travaglia et al., 2011).

Creative thinking strategies that have been found to be useful in helping healthcare professionals deal with constant change include developing personal resilience and the use of mindfulness. Such approaches are outlined in other chapters and so they will not be reiterated here. However, it is worthwhile mentioning the mindfulness technique of 'The Struggle Switch' by Harris (2006), as this would seem to have particular relevance to enabling adaptation to change in healthcare. 'The Struggle Switch' describes how, in life, individuals face many difficulties and challenges that provoke numerous psychological responses, such as the recall of problematic experiences and feelings. Harris (ibid.) explains how the use of 'Acceptance and Commitment Therapy (ACT)' can help deal with these experiences in a more positive way. This is achieved by using a series of value-guided experiential exercises and mindfulness skills.

Opinions on how to deal with change and examples of what has helped to produce positive personal outcomes have been documented by nurses in social media and online blogs. Suggestions have included processes to develop and enhance self-awareness, stress management, personal communication skills, self-esteem and empowerment. It is also apparent that despite the existence of 'burnout' in nursing, many care professionals adjust in a positive way to change and are able to retain their positive views about working in healthcare and their commitment to providing high-quality person-centred care. Indeed, there are many examples of excellent practice despite the pressures of working in contemporary healthcare services.

Additionally, student nurses often describe how highly they value the support of experienced and professional mentors. The author frequently holds reflective discussions with nurse learners during their final management placement. These conversations involve an analysis of learning experiences with different mentors throughout the course and what qualities they would adopt when they become a mentor. What is often espoused is how the students value the mentors who have several years of experience but who have been able to maintain their enthusiasm not only to provide excellent nursing care but also to maintain their commitment to mentor and teach students. How have these mentors been able to retain such commitment after years of care work and how have they avoided burnout or dealt with the high levels of stress? The coping and change strategies employed by these nurses are also cited in online blogs and include being able to maintain a work–life balance, sustain 'meaning' in clinical work, update professional knowledge and competence and continue in their ability to retain value-based care.

Carlson (2017) explores how nurses now have greater autonomy in many aspects of clinical care and, because of this, they can set the schedule for change and act as change agents. Carlson (ibid.) also emphasises that nurses are able to become 'change disrupters'. An example of this is when a nurse observes that an intervention is no longer effective, so it can be 'disrupted' and a new approach initiated. In a comparable manner, nurses have a strong collective voice, and so the culture of an organisation can also be 'disrupted' in a similar way. According to Carlson, the best way of achieving such change and senior management support is by using evidence-based practice, nursing science and common sense. This seems to be a vital assertion because the potential of the nursing workforce as a collective change force appears to have been underutilised by the profession.

Similarly, an eclectic model of good practice in change could also prove to be useful. For, if change can be enabled rather than just managed, then the positive features, principles and experiences of change can be used to reappraise the philosophy of a service by helping to integrate potentially competing forces into a model of good practice. An eclectic paradigm of change is concerned with taking the best parts of each model in order to fit with the uniqueness of change experiences in nursing. Healthcare providers based on social enterprise business models seem to have been particularly successful in this respect and thrive by operating collegiate and staff partnership concepts at all strategic levels.

Conclusion

The level of external scrutiny on nurses is more significant than it has ever been. This chapter has explored how the rate of change and a range of pressures have the potential to cause significant personal stress for nurses. The impact has been ana-lysed from several theoretical perspectives, resulting in the suggestion that constant change has become the norm. It is typical for nurses to feel pressure personally in this context and so strategies that might help the individual deal with continuous change have been described.

References

Brandon, D. (1991) *Innovation without Change? Consumer Power in Psychiatric Services*. Basingstoke: Macmillan Education.

Brooker, D. (2007) *Person-Centred Dementia Care: Making Services Better*. London: Jessica Kingsley Publishers.

Carlson, K. (2017) 'Nurses as disrupters of change', *Nurselife*, 7 June. Available at: www.ausmed.com/articles/nurses-as-disrupters-agents-of-change/ (accessed 19 September 2017).

Carver, C.S. and Scheier, M. (2012) *Perspectives on Personality*. Upper Saddle River, NJ, and London: Pearson.

Chaskalson, M. (2011) *The Mindful Workplace: Developing Resilient Individuals and Resonant Organizations with MBSR*. Oxford: Wiley.

de Silva, D. (2015) *What's Getting in the Way? Barriers to Change in the NHS*. London: The Health Foundation.

Festinger, L. (1962) *A Theory of Cognitive Dissonance*. London: Tavistock Publications.

Harris, R. (2006) 'Embracing your demons: An overview of acceptance and commitment therapy', *Psychotherapy in Australia*, 12 (4): 2–8.

Health Education England (2014) *Literature Review on Nurses Leaving the NHS*. London: Health Education England.

Higgs, J. (2012) *The KLF: Chaos, Magic and the Band who Burned a Million Pounds*. London: Orion.

Hockenbury, D.H. and Hockenbury, S.E. (2006) *Psychology*. New York: Worth.

Kelly, G. (2013) [1959] *A Theory of Personality: Psychology of Personal Constructs*. London: Norton.

Khamisa, N., Oldenburg, B., Peltzer, K. and Illic, D. (2015) 'Work-related stress, burnout, job satisfaction and general health of nurses', *International Journal of Environmental Research and Public Health*, 12: 652–66.

Kitwood, T. (1997) *Dementia Reconsidered: The Person Comes First*. Buckingham: Open University Press.

Kubler-Ross, E. (1969) *On Death and Dying: What the Dying Have to Teach Doctors, Nurses, Clergy, and Their Own Families*. New York: Touchstone.

Lewin, K. and Gold, M. (1999) *The Complete Social Scientist: A Kurt Lewin Reader*. London: American Psychological Association.

Lippitt, R., Westley, B. and Watson, J. (1958) *The Dynamics of Planned Change*. San Diego, CA: Harcourt, Brace and World.

Maslach, C. (1982) *Burnout: The Cost of Caring*. Paramus, NJ: Prentice-Hall.

Mueller, J. (2017) *Creative Change*. Boston, MA: Houghton Mifflin Harcourt.

Office for National Statistics (ONS) (2017) *Deaths Registered in England and Wales* (Series DR) 2015. London: ONS.

Rogers, E.M. (1995) *Diffusion of Innovations*. New York: Free Press.

Sawbridge, Y. and Hewison, A. (2011) 'Time to care? Responding to concerns about poor nursing care'. *HSMC Policy Paper*, 12. Birmingham: Health Services Management Centre, University of Birmingham.

Travaglia, J.D., Thoms, D., Hillman, K., Middleton, S., Hughes. C. and Braithwaite, J. (2011) *Change Management Strategies and Practice Development in Nursing: A Review of the Literature*. Sydney: University of New South Wales.

Welch, J. (2000) *GE Annual Report 2000*. Fairfield: General Electric Company.

Wren, B. (2016) *True Tales of Organisational Life: Using Psychology to Create New Spaces and Have New Conversations at Work*. London: Karnac Books.

3

Nursing

A Profession with Too Many Masters?

Peter J. Martin and Martin Harrison

Chapter aims

- Understand why politics is such an integral component of healthcare.
- Learn to revise our thinking to help us manage (with) the third person in the room.
- Appreciate the destructive nature of battles fought on the ward.
- See nursing as a potential force for positive change.

Introduction

As nurses, it is probably a 'given' that we seek to provide the best quality of care to service users. Nurses are honourable, the media (mostly) tells us so all the time; when we encounter the public, we are told: 'I couldn't do your job, dear.' We are good people. However, in the 2017 Annual National Health Service (NHS) Staff Survey Briefing (NHS Staff Surveys, 2017), only 43 per cent of health service personnel respondents were satisfied with the extent to which their work was valued by their organisation.

In the relationship between nurses and management, the nurse has a 'face', often downtrodden, weary but still caring; in the meanwhile, management is so often characterised as a 'faceless' bureaucracy. In many of the stories that nurses tell everyday about practice, the 'management' is held to be the root of all things bad, the creator of stress and the constrainer of resources.

In its simplistic form, there is an imagined chasm between 'good' nursing and 'bad' management. In this chapter, we will explore the divisiveness of this argument and the potential harm that comes from not 'managing' that shadowy third person, who sits alongside you and the service user.

The Third Man

When we are working with a patient in order to facilitate their recovery, in whatever healthcare setting, it is uncomfortable to acknowledge that there is a political dimension to our interaction. Whether we accept it, or are even aware of it, politics *is* integral to nursing.

Throughout the 1949 film of Graham Greene's *The Third Man*, Harry Lime is a central character but, for much of the film, does not emerge from the murky underworld from which he operates. Lime exerts a great influence on the events recounted in the story, but spends most of the film's duration as an occasional shadow in the background.

For nurses, our 'third man in the room' is the 'politician', who never actually appears but influences events from the shadows. This third person, politician, bureaucrat or manager, represents the non-clinical dimension of our work. When we work with a patient to provide some form of physical intervention or engage through the therapeutic relationship with someone to promote their own recovery from mental illness, we are not alone.

In every decision that we make, however autonomous we may feel it to be, the impact of this political dimension is felt. Our clinical judgement, however person-centred, takes account of available resources, current policy and health and social care diktats. This may be subtle or obvious (see Activity 3.1 for an example).

· ·

Activity 3.1   Reflective Exercise

We wanted to be able to offer our clients a comfortable, quietening environment, where we could work with them to complete a Life-Story Work Book. This is good contemporary practice for people experiencing dementia and we want to be able to incorporate it into our work. But the Trust didn't have the money to decorate the room, so we ended up using this old, drab, single room. It isn't a very inspiring space and the carers particularly have commented on it, saying it reminds them of how hospitals used to look. This isn't helpful with someone who has dementia.

The scenario described above is the type of story that we hear regularly from practitioners. Can you think of some recent examples from your own practice in which you encountered similar problems?

· ·

Of course, you may be feeling that politics has always influenced clinical practice through the exercise of economic control or changes to health policy. Such intrusions are something with which nurses have always had to contend and are a consequence of the organisation of individual nurses into a centrally funded, professional nursing service.

Throughout much of the twentieth century, nursing had a powerful voice and a relatively high degree of autonomy. This autonomy was important when working with a *third person in the room* as it enabled nurses to influence decision-making to the benefit of their patients and, thus, do the best for their patient through delivering compassionate nursing. Arguably, this changed with the introduction of general management into the NHS in the 1980s:

> For some the introduction of general management in the early 1980 was regarded as an attack on both professional autonomy and clinical freedoms. It attracted a predictably hostile reception from both doctors and nurses. (Fatchett, 2013: 245)

Today's health organisations are managing in a difficult environment, balancing a combination of changing patient needs, the scale of the service, economic austerity, patient expectations, monitoring and a growing culture of litigation. Nonetheless, Trust Boards aspire to engage staff and patients in open communication and decision-making in order to deliver services to the maximum benefit of the local community within a finite budget.

In order to communicate through large organisations, some health organisations use Trust Briefing, in-house e-magazines or a number of other strategies to share their 'direction of travel' with the staff team. However, to a junior nurse working in a clinical environment, the decisions of the Trust Board may seem to be made a long way off, and to be puzzling and without a two-way component. The Annual NHS Staff Survey (NHS Staff Surveys, 2017) reported that just one third (33 per cent) of respondents felt that there was good communication between senior management and staff:

> There is compelling evidence that NHS organisations in which staff report that they are engaged and valued deliver better quality care. Superior performance is evident in lower mortality rates and better patient experience. The corollary is that organisations with a disengaged workforce are more likely to deliver care that falls short of acceptable standards. (King's Fund, 2014: 7)

> The contribution of junior doctors and student nurses to the review process was hugely important. They are capable of providing valuable insights, but too many are not being valued or listened to. (Keogh Report, 2013: 12)

There is a growing distance between the decision-making and the bedside; the 'third person in the room' got bigger and the nurse got smaller.

Blurred lines

In every encounter that we have with patients, we make clinical judgements based upon the clinical need of the person before us. However, we are also working in an environment where resources are limited. In a busy healthcare environment, do we, or can we, retain a clear differentiation between judgements informed by clinical need and those informed by resource availability, and thus potentially by our own values?

The majority of nurses work in some form of organised healthcare system. In the UK, these systems may be a sector of the National Health Service, an independent healthcare provider or in the armed forces.

In 1942, the Beveridge Report (Beveridge, 1942) identified the five great evils of the post-war society. These evils were: want, disease, ignorance, squalor and idleness – and the Labour government of the day was committed to working towards reducing each one of them during its term of office. The establishment of the NHS was one response to these evils:

> No society can legitimately call itself civilised if a sick person is denied medical aid because of the lack of means. (Bevan, 1952: 75)

On its establishment, the NHS promised to provide a service to all in need that was free at the point of delivery. Funding for the service was through taxation, which took away the fear of needing to see a doctor but not having the means to pay for the consultation. Despite a difficult, and very well-documented, gestation the NHS was established in 1948.

Whilst the NHS was a unique and human response to managing the health of the nation, there quickly emerged a flaw within the system: health needs were 'infinite', whilst health resources were 'finite'. A year after the NHS's inception, the NHS Amendment Act (1949) paved the way for charges to be made for some services, for example charges for prescriptions were introduced in 1952.

In the NHS in England today, major decisions about the allocation of finite resources are made at NHS England, Clinical Commissioning Groups or around the Board Room table by the Trust Executive Team. However, the impact of budgetary allocation decisions is experienced at the patient interface. It is often left to the nurse to explain to the patient and their carer why there is such a long wait or why specific treatments are not available on the NHS.

The 'infinite' need means that resource-allocation decisions have to be made by health professionals. Part of decision-making means that we have to recognise and

. . . .

Activity 3.2   Reflective Exercise

(1) I know that sometimes we cannot provide the protected time that service users need and this is recorded in their care plans. But, if we haven't got enough staff, then what can we do? We always try and make up for this, though, but it is very tiring.

(2) We had a patient the other day in A&E who presented with a painful shoulder. There were other people around who had been waiting nearly up to the limit. So, when we took him straight through, they were, like, throwing daggers at us; but we knew he needed to be seen quickly.

These two scenarios reflect the types of stories that we hear regularly from practitioners. Can you think of some recent examples from your own practice where you have struggled with how to communicate the impact of a budgetary decision to patients?

. . . .

respond to the moment-by-moment changes to services. Such decisions may mean that someone is deprived of resources if someone else's need is, or becomes, greater. At the frontline of services, these decisions have an immediate and evident impact.

It would be flippant to suggest that a Trust Accountant or Chief Executive do not give any conscious thought to the impact that more stringent budget constraints or actual budget cuts to patient services may have. However, on a spreadsheet, this awareness may not be experienced as keenly as by the nurse confronted with an angry, distressed or despairing patient.

The frontline staff in a clinical setting are often junior, whilst those with greater experience and qualification 'direct' patient care through delegation. In many of the stories that we tell about nursing practice, the senior member of staff so often extols the virtues of 'getting out onto the floor' and engaging with patients. Such statements are often accompanied by a sigh and the observation that, because of the paperwork, this so rarely happens.

Yet, where else, other than at the bedside, should these senior and expert nurses be? Their experience and expertise should be used to lead high standards of care through the direct support of less experienced colleagues. Unfortunately, time for such leadership is channelled into administrative tasks such as staffing rotas, budget management and the production of 'data' in order to evidence the success, or otherwise, of the Trust at meeting arbitrary performance targets.

There have been long-standing public concerns over too many administrators and not enough nurses (Edwards, 2016). Perhaps this is why so many expert nurses are now engaged in 'data entry' rather than championing excellence in nursing care.

We frequently observe that more junior staff and students are often advised to 'learn their trade' by spending time with patients, at the bedside. This seems like excellent practice and a prerequisite for becoming a good nurse, provided that there is adequate teaching, supervision and mentorship available to support the learning process, which is not always the case as reported in *'Raising the Bar: Shape of Caring Report'*: 'work on mentorship has shown that, while students greatly value the support of their mentor, significant variation exists in the quality of mentorship' (Willis, 2015: 46). As a consequence, the group that is often at the forefront of managing the implications of restricted resources is often made up of those who are least prepared and many, newly qualified, who are operating at the level of 'competent' (Benner, 1984).

Into this potent mix we should add the level of activity currently commonplace within healthcare services. Nurses describe themselves as constantly doing something and not having the time to stop and reflect on the quality of care that is being delivered. A range of demographic factors (e.g., age, long-term conditions, increasing population, mental ill health), are all conspiring to increase the acuity of wards, clinics and the communities served by nurses.

When a nurse makes a decision, whether large or small, it needs to be made with the awareness of how the decision is reached. The nurse might ask: 'To what degree has my decision been based on the patient's clinical need and to what degree has the availability of resources been a consideration?' Good decision-making needs to take place in a calm, reflective space, where the judgement can be subject to critical consideration.

There are several models of clinical judgement that have been described (Banning, 2008; Thompson and Dowding, 2002 and others). Importantly, such models focus on clinical decision-making in relation to patient need. However, as we have explored previously, more inexperienced nurses who are working in busy health environments, making decisions under time pressures may confuse the clinical needs of the patient with what can be done within the available resources.

Scenario 3.1   Marlon's Story

Marlon has been working with Lukas, a young man who can be quite volatile because of what the voices he hears in his head are telling him. Over some weeks, Marlon has worked closely with Lukas, helping him to gain more control over his voice-hearing and had built up quite a good therapeutic relationship with him. One thing that Marlon found really worked for Lukas was to be outside kicking a ball around or jogging round the garden when the voices were really bad.

On one shift, Lukas told Marlon that he was struggling as he had lost control of the voices; he asked if they could both go outside for a short while. The ward was really short-staffed; but Marlon also recognised that, considering the distress he was under, Lukas was being very reasonable in his request. Marlon explained the situation and Lukas said that he would wait until Marlon had time to spend with him. Unfortunately, Marlon's shift got busier and there never was enough time or staff on that day to accede to Lukas's request.

Throughout the day, Lukas got more and more distressed, and started to become destructive. The response, in the absence of time to spend with Lukas, was to use PRN medication, which made Lukas a little calmer. The situation left Marlon feeling that he had not delivered good mental health nursing on that shift. This left him feeling despondent and demoralised.

To give you an example of how this works, let us think about a nurse working on a mental health forensic unit. Marlon has recently qualified and is working in an environment in which he is happy (Scenario 3.1).

In this scenario, we see that Lukas's clinical need to be *outside, using up some excess energy* is compromised by available resources, the lack of staff. We have already acknowledged that need is 'infinite' and must be balanced against 'finite' resources. We recognise that just because 'Lukas', or whoever it may be, wants something, it does not mean that it can, or even should, be immediately available.

All the nurses we know are, essentially, pragmatists and know that there will always be exceptional days when resources seriously and adversely impact on care delivery to patients. This has been the same since nursing was first organised into a service. Think about the last outbreak of diarrhoea and vomiting on your ward: nursing continued, it may not have been perfect but nurses worked hard in an attempt to ensure that patients did not suffer. The problem seems to be that the 'exceptional' days are increasingly the 'norm' for many nurses.

The nurse in the scenario above, having experienced too many 'exceptional' days, is beginning to question a basic tenet of mental health nursing, the therapeutic relationship. The therapeutic relationship includes nine constructs: conveying understanding and empathy; accepting individuality; providing support; being there/being available; being genuine; promoting equality; demonstrating respect; maintaining clear boundaries; and having self-awareness (Dzopia and Ahern, 2008). Marlon is aware of what the therapeutic relationship should consist; he will have learned this as a student and will have reflected on the relationship throughout his career. However, what he knows is the right thing to do cannot be achieved; consequently, the compassionate component of nursing remains unattained and the nurse's self-esteem is damaged.

One of Schön's (1983) contentions about much professional education was that it prepared people for a form of practice that only existed in textbooks. In such scenarios, it is all too easy for the nurse to finish the shift feeling an internalised anger, or guilt, that s/he has let the patient down in some way.

So, as in the scenario above, it is the frontline staff who have to work with resource decisions; and it is these frontline staff who are often least equipped to manage the contradictions embedded in these decisions. Such contradictions can be expressed as how much a decision is based on clinical need and how much is a pragmatic recognition of what is possible within stretched resources. The lines between decisions made on clinical need and those based on resource allocation become blurred. Blurred lines are problematic; like a white line on a road in heavy rain, if you can't see it clearly, then there is a danger of crossing the white line into the path of oncoming vehicles.

For an inexperienced nurse who has never known anything different, or for the nurse experiencing too many 'exceptional' days, nursing can become about the 'task' and the 'resource' rather than the person facing you. Nursing risks losing its humanity and becoming just another job:

> If a nurse declines to do these kinds of things for her patient, 'because it is not her business' I should say that nursing was not her calling. I have seen surgical 'sisters', women whose hands were worth to them two or three guineas a week, down upon their knees scouring a room or a hut, because they thought it otherwise not fit for their patients to go into. I am far from wishing nurses to scour. It is a waste of power. But I do say that these women had the true nurse-calling – the good of their sick first and second only the consideration of what it was their place to do – and that women who wait for the housemaids to do this, or for the charwomen to do that, when their patients are suffering, have not the making of a nurse in them. (Nightingale, 1859: 13)

Too Many Masters?

The Nursing and Midwifery Council (NMC) is described as our 'regulatory body' in regulating nurses and midwives and has a very specific role (Table 3.1).

In addition to professional regulation through The Code (NMC, 2015), nurses must be guided by the 6Cs; and all healthcare practitioners in the NHS must be guided by the NHS Constitution, its principles and values (Table 3.2).

Table 3.1 Responsibilities of the NMC

The NMC is responsible for	The NMC is not responsible for
• Regulation of nurses and midwives in England, Wales, Scotland and Northern Ireland	• Regulating hospitals or other healthcare settings
• Protecting the public	• Regulating healthcare assistants
• Setting standards of education, training, conduct and performance	• Representing or campaigning on behalf of nurses and midwives
• Ensuring nurses and midwives are current in terms of skills and knowledge	• Setting levels of staffing
• Ensure nurses uphold our professional standards	
• Undertake investigations into nurses and midwives who fall short of our standards	
• Maintain a register of nurses and midwives allowed to practise in the UK	

Source: NMC (2017a)

Table 3.2 The 6Cs and NHS Values

The 6Cs	NHS Values
• Compassion	• Working together for patients
• Courage	• Respect and dignity
• Commitment	• Commitment to quality of care
• Communication	• Compassion
• Caring	• Improving lives
• Competence	• Everyone counts
(NHS England, 2017a)	(NHS England, 2017b)

If we look at those to whom the nurse has some accountability there are several organisations and individuals (Figure 3.1).

Having too many masters can lead to contradictions and conflicts for nurses. For example, a nurse working on a ward that she considers, in her professional judgement, to have 'inadequate' staffing to meet patient demands, must respond within the terms of the Code:

NMC Code – 16.1 Raise and, if necessary, escalate any concerns you may have about patient or public safety, or the level of care people are receiving in your workplace or any other healthcare setting and use the channels available to you in line with our guidance and your local working practices (NMC, 2015a). If, having taken such action, staffing levels remain unchanged what action

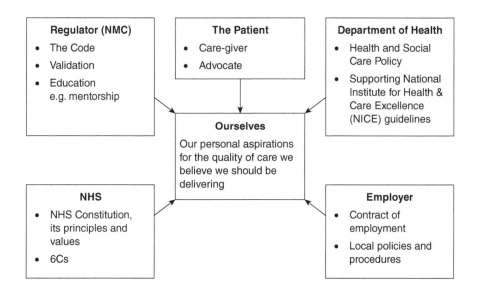

Figure 3.1   Does nursing have too many masters?

can the nurse take considering the NMC (2015b) state that what they are not responsible for includes:

- regulating hospitals or other healthcare settings
- setting levels of staffing

(Reproduced with permission of the Nursing and Midwifery Council.)

We do, of course, recognise the significant role that professional bodies such as the Royal College of Nursing and unions who represent nurses, have played in improving health and social care. The scenario described above serves only to display one of the many apparent contradictions that exist for nurses. For a nurse to have 'too many masters' is stressful but can, at least, be tolerable, provided that they are all working collaboratively toward the same aim. For example, an alteration to an aspect of care delivery may be experienced, on the ground, through: a change in service commissioning arrangements; the arrival of a new policy from the service manager, accompanied by new forms of documentation; and revised good practice guidance from the NMC. However stressful a change may be, there is still a standard of consistent communication to be had when rolling a policy change out.

Inconsistent communication became a problem at the start of 2017, when a leaked memo highlighted a distinct split between orders coming from NHS England to local Trusts and Clinical Commissioning Groups about how to report their individual working conditions to the press. A report in *The Daily Telegraph* by the Health Editor Laura Donnelly summarised the apparent problem in her piece, 'NHS "Spinning" Winter Crisis', exploring the recurring problems that winter illnesses create for the NHS in terms of bed availability and resource usage (2017). The article, slightly sensationalist, suggests that in order to avoid negative publicity, 'local' (Trust) hospital managers were being advised by the 'national' NHS (NHS England) to modulate what was being communicated to the local media about the emerging 'crisis'. This modulation was to be achieved by a cautious use of the language in any official press release. The article cites a memo, reportedly received by senior hospital managers, which seemed to want individual Trusts to play down the crisis, explicitly telling them to avoid language such as 'black alert' – the highest level of emergency.

Whilst it is acknowledged that the article was written for journalistic impact, it exposes a narrowness that we see too much in such reporting of crises in the NHS. This is where the actual experience of managing winter crises by hospital managers, and lower-level members of staff, alongside the immense pressures faced by all, is placed below the need to make a sound bite out of a crisis for public consumption. Indeed, the author may have considered that rather than being purposefully deceptive, the decision to avoid overly emotive terms in press releases was a sensible way to try and create less panic amongst the general public. The problem, however, is that nurses and other health staff are 'the public' also, which is something that those putting out the memo and journalists reporting on the crisis tend to forget.

A nurse working in an A&E department may experience a service under immense stress on a daily basis, and feel that this is not being acknowledged by hospital managers when all they see is the communication of a rather cold, evasive memo. Indeed, the competing narratives underlying the management of winter crises in this country are complex, especially when several bodies are involved in maintaining their own agendas and reputations during them. Managing a service under pressure is demanding but if nurses in that service feel that their managers are not being honest or are failing to acknowledge the conditions under which they are working, then this is devaluing and creates a breakdown of trust. When the dust settled on the reporting of the 2016–17 'NHS Winter Crisis', as it did, perhaps the most lasting impact on our hypothetical but very real nurse working in A&E, was the apprehension that he or she felt about the prospect of the following NHS winter crises to come.

Thus, we have established that nurses, as frontline staff, find themselves managing the mismatch between clinical need and available resources. We find also that the demands placed upon nurses can conflict, leaving the nurse caught between two (or more) 'masters'. All this can leave the compassionate nurse feeling that they are operating in a battlefield.

Battlefield ward

Currently, in the UK, there are growing pressures on the healthcare system. The source of this pressure can be attributed to a combination of economic austerity and associated service redesign, an increasingly elderly population and an increase in long-term illness conditions.

The combination of high levels of activity and a sense of impending crises has led to what we can describe as a state of 'Normalised Chaos'. In 'Normalised Chaos', the 'exceptional days' described earlier become normalised and behaviours associated with crises also become commonplace. In Case Study 3.1, Jenny offers a view of the tensions in contemporary healthcare. Jenny has been a nurse for 32 years and is currently a senior clinical manager, working in an acute sector in an NHS Trust in England.

Case Study 3.1   Jenny's Story

Sadly, there is conflict most days within the acute sector of a general hospital. Patients attend the Emergency Department. They are sick, whether physically or mentally. The hospitals are struggling with inadequate space to care for the patients they already have. There are issues with social care beds. The population is getting older and we have the ability to perform more surgery, more investigations and more interventions. There are targets to meet, not only within the Emergency Department but within the ambulance service, within radiology and pathology and also within surgical waiting lists.

So, where does this leave our patient? Politically, the patient must travel through the Emergency Department within four hours from the moment they are booked in by the reception staff either to discharge or admission to a ward.

Professionally, I want to give the best care possible to that patient. Yes, that does involve transferring the patient to the most appropriate setting in a timely manner but it also means ensuring that I have given the care that the patient deserves. It also means that I have completed the observations regularly and I have given all the treatment that the patient needs. Personally, I want the patient to receive the care that I would want given to my family and loved ones. Moreover, I want to be able to tell the patient's relatives that I have been able to do exactly that:

- My nursing head tells me that I will care for the patient as I have been taught and how I know is right.

- My personal head tells me that I will be the patient's advocate and give the care that the patient deserves.

- My managers expect me to justify why the patient is still within the Emergency Department after four hours.

Critical reflection (Brookfield, 1995) may help us to understand and make sense of what is occurring. The subtext of Jenny's account is that, despite seniority, she exists in a world over which she exercises minimal control and that consists of ever increasing activity, underpinned by conflict and struggle.

The way in which we think is informed by the assumptions we hold about the world around us (Brookfield, 1995). The simplest and most easily accessible of these assumptions are causal and we must understand causal assumptions in order to uncover other, more deeply held, assumptions. Causal assumptions are often the link between 'cause and effect'. In Jenny's story in Case Study 3.1, we can outline the causal assumptions that she holds and how they are constructed:

- If I meet the targets set for me as my employer demands, then I will have done my job well.
- If I treat the patient as my personal philosophy demands, then I will have done my job well.
- If I advocate for my patients, as the NMC Code (NMC, 2015a) paragraph 3.4 dictates, then I will have done my job well.

An appreciation of the contextual background of assumptions will also help us to understand why we hold them. The context of Jenny's story includes:

- Austerity, underpinned by economic recession, is a policy to reduce deficits by reducing the budgets of many public services. Whilst healthcare has, to a larger extent, been protected, in practice, cuts to associated services have adversely impacted on healthcare. For example, cuts in social care have amplified problems of bed usage in the NHS and the derogatory term 'bed-blockers' has re-emerged.
- Generically applied political imperatives in relation to throughput (e.g., 4-hour A&E wait) driven by expediency rather than patient need.
- Awareness of the consequences of failure to meet political demands. For example, by exceeding the 4-hour target, a department is described as 'breaching'. Synonyms for breaching include, 'breaking', 'rupturing', 'contravening' and 'violating'. Such terms carry with them an air of threat.
- A vocational person-centred attitude to work, to do the best for my patients.

Having identified assumptions and considered context, Brookfield (1995) encourages us to *think outside the box*. Jenny's story may appear intractable: What more can she do to change the situation in which she finds herself? How can she look at this differently?

Critical reflection may not help resolve the situation; after all, without control of the resources, Jenny cannot increase her staff complement nor create new bed spaces. So, what is the point of thinking about the situation in a critical way?

Critical reflection might help us understand that we are not actually fighting the third person but ourselves. The third person in the room is a chimera, consisting of what we believe we *should* be doing. Spending time becoming stressed about what we should be doing if we were given the resources is, ultimately, fruitless. It can only end up leaving us feeling demoralised, demotivated and disempowered.

Locus of control

What can be done? It is only by trying to make sense of what is happening that we will be able to see more clearly what is actually happening. Nursing appears to be stuck between two conflicting 'images': an external and an internal view. First, the view that is held by others of the caring, compassionate human being, and, second, the view that we hold of ourselves as subjugated, disempowered workers.

The 'Locus of Control' originally described by Rotter (1954) but extensively developed by others, is a way in which we can look at nursing. Currently, there seems to be a dominant externalised locus of control, as in Jenny's story, where she feels powerless within an increasingly chaotic system. A stronger internal locus of control can help us feel ownership for what we can control rather than being self-critical about things that we do not control.

The payback for the emotional labour (Hochschild, 1983) that nurses put into their work is the satisfaction of delivering the best nursing care that is possible at that moment. Maybe it is at 'that moment' that Watson's (1999) human-to-human transaction occurs, the *phenomenological field* from which both the person and the nurse benefit. Maybe it is at that moment, when we are being the best we can be, that we should stop and reflect rather than when we are staring into our coffee cup on a short-lived break from the ward.

In an article on the 'Normalization of Deviance' in health systems, Banja (2010) offers some more practical advice. In his conclusion, he asserts that a fundamental commitment to patient safety can be developed through five principles:

- *Paying attention to weak signals*: Making sure that you always communicate clearly and unambiguously. For example, we might express to colleagues and managers that, 'There are not enough single rooms to give respectful and dignified nursing care.' Perhaps, in the future, we should be saying more clearly, 'We need more single rooms in order for nurses to give respectful and dignified nursing care.' Saying it once, twice or even thrice may not have an impact, but if we 690, 773 (all nurses registered on NMC in March 2017, see NMC, 2017b) nurses all started speaking more assertively and consistently about where things need to be improved, maybe we could be heard.

- *Resisting the urge to be unreasonably optimistic*: The current situation in healthcare is unlikely to improve significantly over the next few years. By simply acknowledging that this is the world in which we exist, we run the risk of assuming that we will 'get through' and we become complacent of the disaster around the corner. We need to be vigilant and avoid assuming that everything will be alright.

- *Teaching employees how to conduct emotionally uncomfortable conversations*: This principle, for the purposes of this chapter, can be understood as the importance of sharing the skills and knowledge that allow some people to speak up assertively when they encounter bad practices.

- *Nurses feeling safe in speaking up*: Using organisational procedures and the NMC's guidance on speaking out to bring deficiencies to the attention of managers promptly, unambiguously and unemotionally.

- *Realising that oversight and monitoring for rule compliance are never-ending*: The final principle concerns the nature of risk within the health organisation. Banja argues that health organisations are complex and that risk is ever present. An internalised locus of control can help us be more aware of the risks around us, for ourselves, our colleagues and our patients.

Conclusion

We know that nursing work intrinsically involves high levels of emotional labour (Hochschild, 1983). As nurses, we are expected, repeatedly, to deal with emotionally draining activities and then to move on to the next activity without allowing our stress and distress to show. In one moment, we are managing an antagonistic, angry individual, in the next a tearful, bereaved older adult. In Jenny's story, she is working with the existing emotional labour of the job and having to manage the additional pressures that targets and workload impose.

It is impossible not to hypothesise that this pressure will have an impact on the health and well-being of nurses. Anecdotally, the authors are aware of many nurses in senior positions who are looking for early retirement or, ironically, some who are looking for jobs in education, which they perceive as an easier, more autonomous, option. The irony here is, of course, that in moving to education without addressing the problems of practice, one is simply creating a new body of nurses to face the same predicaments. This can begin to feel, at best, like Schön's (1983) critique of professional education or, at worst, like making 'cannon fodder'.

References

Banja, J. (2010) 'The normalization of deviance in healthcare delivery', *Business Horizons*, 53: 139–48.

Banning, M. (2008) 'A review of clinical decision making: Models and current research', *Journal of Clinical Nursing*, 17: 187–9.

Benner, P. (1984) *From Novice to Expert*. Boston, MA: Addison-Wesley.

Bevan, N. (1952) *In Place of Fear*. London: Heinnemann.

Beveridge, W. (1942) *Social Insurance and Allied Services* (*The Beveridge Report*), Cmd 6404. London: HMSO.

Brookfield, S. (1995) *Becoming a Critically Reflective Teacher*. San Francisco, CA: Jossey-Bass.

Donnelly, L. (2017) 'NHS "spinning" winter crisis', *The Daily Telegraph*, 7 January. Available at: www.pressreader.com/uk/the-daily-telegraph/20170107/281487866030333 (accessed January 2017).

Dzopia, F. and Ahern, K. (2008) 'What makes a quality therapeutic relationship in psychiatric/ mental health nursing: A review of the research literature', *Internet Journal of Advanced Nursing Practice*, 10.

Edwards, N. (2016) 'Wasteful, too many chiefs: Five myths about the NHS we need to dispel', *The Guardian*, 26 January. Available at: www.theguardian.com/society/commentisfree/2016/ jan/26/five-myths-nhs-health-service (accessed April 2017).

Fatchett, A. (2013) *Social Policy for Nurses*. Cambridge: Polity Press.

Hochschild, A.R. (1983) *The Managed Heart: Commercialisation of Human Feeling*. Berkeley, CA: University of California Press.

Keogh, B. (2013) *Review into the Quality of Care and Treatment Provided by 14 Hospital Trusts in England: Overview Report*. London: Department of Health.

King's Fund (2014) *Improving NHS Care by Engaging Staff and Devolving Decision-Making*. London: King's Fund.

NHS England (2017a) 'The 6Cs'. Available at: www.england.nhs.uk/leadingchange/about/the-6cs/ (accessed December 2017).

NHS England (2017b) 'NHS values in action and making a difference', News, 11 February. Available at: www.england.nhs.uk/2014/02/nhs-values-in-action/ (accessed December 2017).

NHS Staff Surveys (2017) 'Briefing note: Issues highlighted by the 2016 NHS Staff Survey in England', 7 March. Available at: www.nhsstaffsurveys.com/Caches/Files/20170306_ST16_National%20Briefing_v6.0.pdf (accessed April 2017).

Nightingale, F. (1859) *Notes on Nursing: What It is and What It is Not*. London: Harrison. Facsimile edition (1946) published by Edward Stern & Co Philadelphia.

Nursing and Midwifery Council (NMC) (2015a) The Code: Professional Standards of Practice and Behaviour for Nurses and Midwives. London: NMC. Available at: www.nmc.org.uk/globalassets/sitedocuments/nmc-publications/nmc-code.pdf accessed December 2017).

NMC (2015b) *Our Role*. Available at: www.nmc.org.uk/about-us/our-role/ (accessed 12 March 2018).

NMC (2017a) '*Our role*: What we do'. Available at: www.nmc.org.uk/about-us/our-role/ (accessed December 2017).

NMC (2017b) *The NMC Register 2012/13–2016/17*. London: NMC.

Rotter, J.B. (1954) *Social Learning and Clinical Psychology*. New York: Prentice-Hall.

Schön, D. (1983) *The Reflective Practitioner: How Professionals Think in Action*. New York: Basic Books.

Thompson, C. and Dowding, D. (2002) *Clinical Decision-Making and Judgement in Nursing*. London: Churchill Livingstone.

Watson, J. (1999) *Nursing: Human Science and Human Care National League for Nursing*. London: Jones and Bartlett.

Willis, P. (2015) '*Raising the Bar: Shape of Caring*': A Review of the Future Education and Training of Registered Nurses and Care Assistants. London: Health Education England.

4

Reconnecting with your Nursing Values

Cathy Constable

We learn from one another how to be human by identifying ourselves with others, finding their dilemmas in ourselves. What we all learn from it is self-knowledge. The self we learn about ... is every self. IT is universal – the human self. We learn to recognize ourselves in others ... (it) keeps alive our common humanity and avoids reducing self or other to the moral status of object. (Watson, 1988: 59–60)

Chapter aims

- Understand what we mean by values.
- Evaluate why you chose nursing.
- Consider professional socialisation and role conflict.
- Manage the conflict between demonstrating core values and the challenges of the work environment.

Introduction

The first three chapters of the book discuss the external working environment in nursing and why working in healthcare can be so stressful and demanding of its staff. Chapter 1 explores 'the stress of it all' and the difficulties that staff face in working in extremely busy, ever changing environments with competing demands. In such circumstances, we know that daily struggles arise over limited resources.

There is a human tendency to look back on the past through rose-tinted spectacles as though there were a 'golden age' of the NHS. It has always been busy with services in high demand and with nurses having to cope with limited and finite resources from the beginning.

The next four chapters explore how we personally cope with working in these environments. Battles are fought externally but also internally within us as we may feel conflict between the values that drive us to be excellent competent nurses, competing demands of the organisation and its values (which may or may not match ours) and the reality of the busy, changing work environment. Often, this leaves us feeling as though there is a dissonance or conflict between our real self and what our personal and professional values guide us to do when we are confronted with making difficult and complex clinical decisions. Organisation and Trusts advocate idealistic values but staff feel the frustration if they are not translated into practice. This difficulty in not being able to be authentic and 'ourselves' is stressful and anxiety-provoking on a personal level and, when added to the emotional labour of nursing, can lead to feelings of exhaustion and burnout with reduced job satisfaction (Stacey et al., 2011; Price, 2009).

This chapter aims to help you to explore how to identify and hold on to your personal and professional values, with the goal of increasing personal resilience and role satisfaction and creating more control over your worklife. It is important to point out that when offering advice on how to cope in difficult circumstances, the onus is often put on the individual rather than on how the organisation is functioning. In this way, we may feel that we are to blame and we may feel guilty in that, in some way, we are personally failing to cope. We may be failing to cope but we are failing to cope in difficult circumstances.

The emphasis in this chapter is on the unprecedented financial and operational challenges that the NHS is going through. It can be a difficult place for all to work in at times and, therefore, exploring these issues will help you to cope on a personal level rather than ask you to change the organisation. However, building your resilience will have an impact on how you work, your role in a team and, therefore, could have a positive impact on your working environment and, in turn, on the environment in which you care for your patients and service users. As Ballatt and Campling point out, 'self-interest and the interests of others are bound together' (2014: 5).

'Why do you want to be a nurse?'

We have all chosen nursing as a career for different reasons. Think back to how you answered that dreaded question at interview: 'So, why do you want to be a nurse?' or 'What qualities do you have to be a nurse?' The truth is that there are many reasons why. The answers below come from a sample of email poll responses among colleagues and students.

Why I Chose Nursing

'Nursing was not my first choice of career and did not expect to stay in this profession for as long as I have. I was always of the view that it would be a stopgap until I found something else that I was more suited to. Over thirty years later, I am still here. I can't think of any other job that I can or would want to do. For me, the turning point was training as a mental health nurse after being a registered adult nurse. I found that here was something that was interesting, where being with people, listening and learning from the people that I cared for was what made a difference, and realising that understanding the person's concerns needed to be done within the context of their biopsychosocial being.'

Amanda, Mental Health Nurse

'I am driven by contributing towards the good of society, I want to feel that I am 'doing good'. It's not a desire to change the world, or cure anybody, just to make inevitable suffering a little more bearable. Seeing people progressing gives me joy and fulfilment.'

Natalie, Student Mental Health Nurse

'I could also quote, 'I wanted to make a difference' by becoming a Nurse, I suppose this isn't entirely true. Yes, I am a caring person and enjoy being around people, helping them, although my real passion is patho-physiology and human sciences, knowing how the body reacts in illness or in a critical health situation; promoting health and well-being to someone who needs support to maintain a quality of life.'

Susanna, Student Adult Nurse

'I became a nurse due to several influences. I was brought up learning the values of caring and compassion and was expected to uphold these. I knew that I wanted a career in the Humanities, but wasn't sure which of the subjects. I also enjoyed Horticulture which is something that I had also considered. I became aware of how Horticulture was being used as therapy for people with mental health issues and gave that some thought. I then worked in a hospital where horticulture and other occupations were used as therapy. These approaches seemed to have very good outcomes and it confirmed to me that I could combine two interests in my career. I haven't looked back since.'

Thomas, Mental Health Nurse

Values

If I were to ask you what are the important core values in nursing, what would you say? Hopefully, you have been well schooled in current nursing issues and can cite the 6Cs – compassion, care, courage, commitment, communication and competence, as described by the Chief Nursing Officer in *Compassion in Practice* (Cummings and Bennett, 2012). Some others may be integrity, kindness, trustworthiness, diversity and tolerance. You can probably also add some of your own, based on your experiences in life and in nursing.

Who chooses the values that we work within? How do we know they that are 'right'?

The NHS Constitution is based on shared values that patients, the public and staff have developed collaboratively in order to help inspire passion in the NHS and it should underpin everything that it does (NHS, 2015). The Constitution highlights the importance of shared values and staff at all levels, working together to achieve shared aspirations.

The NHS Constitution (2015)

The NHS Constitution establishes the principles and values of the NHS in England. It sets out rights to which patients, public and staff are entitled, and pledges that the NHS is committed to achieve, together with responsibilities, which the public, patients and staff owe to one another in order to ensure that the NHS operates fairly and effectively.

In brief, these values are:

Working together for patients.

Respect and dignity.

Commitment to quality of care.

Compassion.

Improving lives.

Everyone counts.

These values are also echoed and enshrined in the Nursing and Midwifery Code (NMC, 2015), which outlines the values and standards that all nurses and midwives must work to and demonstrate in their practice.

Holt (in Sellman and Snelling, 2017: 27) describes The Code as 'prescriptive', in that it tells registrants what to do. The Code outlines the minimum standards to which nurses need to work. Holt goes on to argue whether or not The Code provides guidance on ethical practice and that this is open to debate. The NMC expects us to act in the best interest of patients and how we do this is left to the nurse to decide. With an acceptance of the limitations of working within codes, it is a useful exercise to revisit what our internal 'codes' are with regards to nursing. This can give us a benchmark that we can revisit when we need to. What values did you bring to nursing and which ones have developed during training and beyond?

I invite you to carry out the mindfulness exercise (written by Caroline Barratt at the University of Essex, 2017) in Activity 4.1, with the aim of thinking about why you wanted to be a nurse. To do this, we want you to contemplate four different questions. Hopefully, this exercise will help you to reconnect with your core values.

....

Activity 4.1   Mindfulness Exercise

To start the activity, find a space where you feel safe and won't be interrupted. Close your eyes for a few moments, take several deeper breaths, gathering your attention and bringing it to the task at hand.

On opening your eyes, read the first question. Close your eyes again for approximately five minutes and see what arises in response to the question. There is no right or wrong answer to any of the questions. When a response arises, notice it and then let it go and come back to sitting quietly with the question.

After five minutes of contemplating the first question, open your eyes and make a few notes about what arose for you.

Repeat this for all four questions below.

If you find it difficult to sit quietly, you may want to use 'free writing' as a way of responding to each question. This method involves reading the question and then writing continuously for three minutes without filtering what you write. If you feel as though you have nothing to write, then simply write, 'I can't think of anything to write,' until further words come. You will not share this with anyone else, so there is no need for censorship.

Both methods facilitate a deeper exploration of the questions – they help us to go beyond our intellectual mind and what we think is the 'correct' answer. Maintaining an attitude of curiosity and openness is important.

Questions:

1.   Why am I a nurse?
2.   What effect do I want my nursing to have on me?
3.   What effect do I want my nursing to have on my patients?
4.   What effect do I want my nursing to have on the world around me?

....

What functions do values perform?

Pattison and Thomas (2010) suggest that values can be thought of as a framework that helps us to understand the world and to guide our behaviour, attitudes and actions. They write about how the radical nature of change in the NHS and between professions over recent years has led to an increase in 'value-talk' in an attempt to make sense of changes and their worth. You may have heard of the terms 'values-based recruitment', 'values-based curriculum' and 'values-based practice'.

Value Functions

- Values legitimise action and organisational arrangements.

- Values help coordinate actions.

- Values can be used to discipline/manage people.

- Values justify change and resistance to change.

- Values help create and consolidate identity.

Source: Pattison and Thomas (2010: 239)

Whilst professional codes give us direction and boundaries within our roles and professions, Francis (2013) points out that there are many different professional codes being adhered to in the NHS, and this can have an impact on the consistency of culture within the NHS. He argues that this can potentially lead to the separation of culture identity within professions.

Excerpt From Report of the Mid Staffordshire NHS Foundation Trust Public Inquiry (2013)

A consistent culture producing the best chance for all patients to be treated in accordance with acceptable fundamental standards of safety and quality requires the NHS and all who work in it to develop and adhere to a common set of standards and values. There are many sources from which such values can be drawn and defined already, but they have been developed from the perspective of individual professions or groups of staff. Many of them derive from professional regulators and have disciplinary connotations. While this may be inevitable, it does mean that they are not sufficient to produce an overall culture shared by all in the healthcare community. Disciplinary codes are necessary but are more likely to be regarded as something to comply with rather than something to be owned and lived by. (Francis, 2013: vol. 3, p. 1400)

Reproduced with permission under the terms of the Open Government License.

Francis goes on to advocate that: 'All staff need to be made part of an overall NHS culture of which they can be proud and identify with. The challenge is to work out how to achieve this' (ibid.: 1400). The Francis Report, of course, led to an internal and external examination of the role of values in the NHS.

Much has been written about the challenges in defining what caring is and what nurses 'do' and this is ongoing (Sellman, 2011; Watson, 2012). One could argue that this is inevitable, as the nursing role should change with the ongoing needs of society. However, this can make it difficult to have a strong, coherent voice, with confident values that define occupational boundaries. The Chief Nursing Officer's report specifically on the role of mental health nurses, *From Values to Action* (Department of Health, 2006), attempted to modernise the mental health nursing profession and advocated the use of recovery-base values in order to promote social inclusion and individualised care based on therapeutic collaborative relationships between service user and nurse.

However, a decade on, and the most recent inquiry into the role of mental health nurses, *Foundation of Nursing Studies* (Butterworth and Shaw, 2017), warns that the mental health nursing profession is still grappling with its identity and ability to answer the question, 'What do mental health nurses do?', in an assertive and consistent way, and the role is potentially at risk of being incorporated into a more generic nurse role. They suggest that mental health nurses take for granted their psychosocial and interpersonal skills and need to be more confident of their work in these areas in order to secure their unique role. Part of this confidence is in being aware of the personal and professional values that drive us in our work.

Diverse understanding of what values mean

So, we have the NMC Code, the NHS Charter, the 6Cs and our employers' set of values to guide our work. Of course, people are diverse and our values can differ hugely. What may be of importance to me, may not be important to you. So, how do we choose what the right values for healthcare are? Even if we agree on a value – i.e., compassion – my understanding of what compassion is for me may not relate to your understanding of it for you. Working with service users and colleagues also with differing cultural views can be complicated in healthcare decision-making, as illustrated by Sally's experience:

'Nursing can be difficult when you find it hard to agree with what the patients want. I remember when I was a student on my community placement, I went to see an older lady who had a terminal illness. Being compassionate to me would have been to make sure she had good pain relief but she kept refusing it despite the family and myself trying to encourage her to have it as she was in great pain. She said she was afraid that she would lose control of her bodily functions. She felt it would be more compassionate to be 'allowed' to remain in control so she could die with dignity. I could see what she meant but I found it very difficult for her and her husband. I remember speaking to my mentor and she said we needed to respect her wishes. We talked about how complicated it all is and that you have to make sure, as a nurse, you can balance everything up in the patient's best interest. It's still not easy.'

Sally, Adult Nurse

Fulford describes values-based practice as: 'the theory and skills base for effective healthcare decision-making where different (and hence potentially conflicting) values are in play' (2004: 16). So, while we have the NMC Code and NHS Constitution to guide us, Woodbridge and Fulford (2005) agree that frameworks of values can differ and potentially seem in conflict with one another.

Values-Based Practice

In values-based practice, these differences in codes, far from being grounds for conflict, provide a balance of different value perspectives which allow decisions to be appropriately matched to the individual values of the particular service user affected by a given decision. Since the codes themselves cannot determine exactly how we can strike a balance, values-based practice provides a theory and a set of skills for turning the different values expressed by different codes from a source of conflict into a positive resource for balanced decision making. (Woodbridge and Fulford, 2005: 57)

© The Sainsbury Centre for Mental Health 2004.

Professional socialisation

Values have an influence on how we act as professionals and help guide the development of professional identity (Woodbridge and Fulford, 2005). This is especially true for student nurses and those who are newly qualified. We often hear from our students that they experience 'reality shock' when they go out on placement and I am sure that all nurses reading this can identify with that feeling. The notion of the theory–practice gap remains. Students can feel torn by the idealisms that they are encouraged to think and write about at university and what they experience on busy placements.

Exploring the impact of professional socialisation on ourselves may give us some clues as to what values are important to us. The concept of professional socialisation is important when thinking about the values that we have. Like it or not, we have all been professionally socialised into nursing! A literature review by Dinmohammadi et al. cites that there are many definitions of what professional socialisation is, 'most of which describe it as the process of internalising and developing a professional identity through the acquisition of knowledge, skills, attitudes, beliefs, values, norms, and ethical standards in order to fulfill a professional role' (2013: 27). However, we also come into nursing with values as voiced by some of the answers of staff and students in Activity 4.2.

Research by Stacey et al. (2011: 22) demonstrated that nurses came into the profession with values consistent with using a person-centred approach and with the values advocated by the NMC and governing bodies. They concluded that nurses were aware of the dissonance that can occur when there is a conflict between their values and the limitations of the workplace and noted that they responded through one of the following:

- *Acceptance*: Continuing to work within the constraints despite experiencing personal conflict.
- *Rejection*: Either leaving or thinking about it.
- *Innovation*: Challenging preconceived workplace beliefs and working to initiate change.

Conversely, we can all remember working with staff whose work practices we would not want to emulate. Interestingly, the research by Stacey et al. (2011) found that participants did not internalise practice that did not reflect their own values. A more recent study by Traynor and Buus (2016) echoes how student nurses tend to identify with qualified nurses who reflect their positive values and they work hard not to be influenced by nurses whom they perceive as 'bad'.

. . . .

Activity 4.2   Positive Role Models

Through experience and professional socialisation, values can change. Think back to when you had an excellent mentor or worked with an outstanding role model and thought, 'This is the way I want to be':

- What was it about them that you admired?
- What values and characteristics did you want to internalise and emulate and why?
- Have you ever asked for feedback from a student whom you are mentoring or a colleague?

It may be that you could also 'identify' with them and had similar values. Indeed, may be *you* are one of those excellent mentors or role models!

. . . .

The Concept of the 'Wounded Healer' in Nursing

> Nobody can meddle with fire or poison without being affected in some vulnerable spot; for the true physician does not stand outside his work but always in the thick of it. (Jung, 1977: 5)

Is there another, more personal, way in which to think about why you came into nursing? What is it about caring that appeals to you? What benefit is there for you in caring for people? Many nurses will talk openly about why they became a nurse and cite their personal experiences with physical illness or mental health issues that have involved relatives or themselves. They may have chosen an area of work for a reason, e.g. working in palliative care because of a family experience of cancer. This can often be a very positive driving force if it is acknowledged and needs are met. However, psychoanalytic theory suggests that some people may also unconsciously seek ways in which to repair previously unresolved past difficult or traumatic experiences. The concept of the the 'wounded healer' is widely discussed in counselling and psychotherapy literature (Sedgwick, 1994), and has much to offer nursing in our attempts to understand our motivation to undertake our roles.

Ballatt and Campling (2014) warn that, while working in healthcare can offer an opportunity for reparation and healing, often the opposite may be true. If the unconscious motivation is to heal a sick family member, when patients do not get better, we may feel guilt and other emotions such as anger and sadness and feel overwhelmed by an attempt to work harder in order to achieve their impossible goal. It becomes a vicious circle, if we are not able or do not have the time to reflect on why we might feel like we do.

McClendon (2005: 8) discusses how she uses Watson's caring–healing theory of nursing to help her understand the cognitive dissonance that she felt when split between the two nursing worlds of practice and academia. She believes that 'this fundamental disconnect wounds many nurses' and this contributes to workplace tensions. She cites Watson:

> The notion of health professionals as wounded healers is acknowledged as part of necessary growth called forth within this theory/philosophy. Caring does signify healing self and others. The more caring there is, the more self-healing and vice versa. Nursing is a lifetime of growth, health and healing. (Watson, 2001: 348)

If we explore the 'wounded healer' in ourselves, it may give us clues as to why we feel like we do in times of stress. Niven (2008) uses the work of Nouwen to encourage us to acknowledge our own 'wounds', reflect on them and accept them as part of the human condition. Making sense of our lives can help expand our understanding of the human condition. We can then use this knowledge as a compassionate resource in helping us to relate to others. Gilbert and Stickley (2012) discuss the positive experiences of students who had experienced mental health problems and felt that this helped them relate to their patients. However, they highlight the importance of maintaining professional boundaries.

Exploring Your Own 'Wounds' in a Safe Environment

- You may choose the process of reflection as described in Chapter 7 in order to explore your reactions to events.

- You may decide that you want to use counselling as an opportunity to explore your inner self and make some sense of how this can help you at work.

(Continued)

(Continued)

- If you can access supervision at work, this may be a comfortable space in which you can explore how better to cope with how you feel at work.

- Chapter 5 on Mindfulness may give you some ideas of how to use this practice to reflect on difficult feelings.

Coping with stress in a healthcare environment: A case study

Below is a transcript of a conversation that I had with a ward manager, Ben, about his values and how he manages to cope with working in a busy inpatient environment. Many of the themes discussed in this chapter are evident in Ben's worklife:

Cathy: What are the kinds of values that you think you bring into nursing?

Ben: My parents were foster parents, so we would have emergency foster children coming into the house who had a lot of emotional problems, so there have always been caring roles around with my Mum and Dad, so I've grown up with those values. Helping people that have a less fortunate background than myself. I have been quite fortunate, so I guess there is something about the gift that I have had in life and helping others that haven't been so lucky.

Cathy: Are there any other values that you have that you can think of?

Ben: Doing the best for people. I'm a big believer if we struggle with people, for example if you work in an acute unit and I can feel myself getting a bit angry or frustrated – have those conversations with colleagues and look at why the person is here. And, also, if that was somebody in your family, how would you want them to be treated in that situation. Because, otherwise, you can go down the road of being burnt out and stressed.

Cathy: So, what happens to you, what do you do at that point when you experience that frustration?

Ben: I've probably been a reflector all my life and not realised until I came into nursing. Nursing has given me the wording of what it was. I think I reflect a lot on action and when I am doing care interventions, I am constantly thinking about 'Is this good quality care?' before it escalates to not consciously providing bad care but going down that route. I think in terms of looking after me, so, for example, making sure I have lunch and trying to do a bit of mindfulness in my lunch break. I've got a guided meditation app I use. Just five minutes at lunch, if I remember!

  (Points to his white board where he has written some notes.) I have got this as well. Whereas I used to go home and it takes me half an hour to get

home I use that time to reflect on everything and mentally reprocess. But there were times when I was still getting home and still feeling anxious and angry. I have my life outside work and it was still impacting on that, so, when I have time, I write things down, sort of 'dumping it at work'. There is something about me being able to write it on the board and just leave it. It may not completely work all the time but it is part of the process and helps.

Cathy: How do you cope on stressful days?

Ben: When I go home, I have got a family, so I just distract myself with them. If I'm having a stressful day and I get home, it's probably for a couple of hours but by the time I've slept and come back in, I feel more refreshed and more able to deal with the challenges of the previous day. There is something about sleep, so me and my partner do guided meditation at night sometimes if we can't sleep, and she enjoys it as well. It's all that sort of self-care stuff.

Cathy: So, you are good at self-care?

Ben: Goodish … ! (Laughs.)

Cathy: So, in terms of your management role, is there anything that you implement with the team to try and keep morale up? I guess it is as busy here as everywhere.

Ben: Yes, everywhere is busy – just different sorts of busy. Reflection is a big thing here, so, when I took the job, we had a team-building day which was the foundations of making the 'roots' with staff, then I've tried to implement reflection, so I'll spend a period of time when I've come in and ask what went well, what didn't go well and what would you do differently next time?

Cathy: Do you do this in handover?

Ben: Yes, sometimes. I'm still working on when it fits best in the work in the ward because you have to remember it's not about what I want, it's about what the team want. So, I am trying to get it into handover but there is also something about being an observer, about what's going on at times. There have been shifts that are possibly going down the avenue of tasks not getting done, potential for incidences and lack of communication, so I will stop and grab people and say, 'You are in charge. Can you tell me what's happening, what's not working well, what are you going to do about it?' It is just to help read, to refocus. They can probably see it themselves that things are heading the wrong way and maybe feeling a bit frustrated. Having that ability just to stop and replan because there is no reason why we can't change direction.

Cathy: I am interested in how we value-check ourselves in the line of fire, if that makes sense: How do you know you're doing the right thing?

Ben: Yes, it's about reflecting and about the feedback you get from relatives and feedback from staff. So, a big thing I tried to build in on the team-building day is about people being able to give feedback as a practitioner. So, I can get feedback on action and provide a rationale for something I'm doing that somebody else isn't sure about. So, that is also a check that I am doing the right thing. Being able to have an open and honest conversation – it keeps me in check and keeps the patient safe. So, we get feedback from service users about our interventions, for example, a reduction in distress. We can also get feedback from relatives and other colleagues about how they perceive the service user.

Cathy: I think that is part of the stress of nursing because we want to come in and help people but if the environment isn't conducive for us to be able to do that, for us personally it can be a struggle?

Ben: I think that we get too bogged down in everything that is going on and we forget the little things. So, we have had to support a very distressed lady today, who was very unhappy with us but actually there was a bit where we were able to give her a drink because she was thirsty. She had been swearing and was being quite aggressive and that's not her but we have managed to do something positive for her, the simple things of giving painkillers to somebody to make them more comfortable. The whole shift might have been terrible but, actually, you've been able to help nourish somebody.

Cathy: Do you feel your values match those of the organisation?

Ben: Not always but it's about giving the organisation feedback. I think I'm in a recognised position where I can escalate my concerns and be listened to. There was an example the other week: the service manager wanted the nursing staff to do another audit and I said, actually, 'Could you get the admin to do this?' A decision hasn't been made yet and it may be that we have to do it but I've still been able to advocate for my staff. I went to university to care for people not to be an auditor, not to fill out paperwork. It is about maintaining that value in your head that you come here to care and being able to say, actually, that's enough, there are other people that can do X,Y and Z.

Cathy: The biggest complaint we get from our newly qualified students is that they don't have time to care, they don't have time to do one-to-one time or therapy.

Ben: Yes, I do think we have gone the other way, so, a colleague of mine, she was telling me when she came into nursing there were lots of nurses and you had five staff on the ward – four nurses and one Health Care Assistant (HCA) – and the nurses were out on the wards. Now, we are HCA top-heavy. They can still help us with our paperwork, bed statements, etc., but I need you (qualified staff) to go out and provide a high-level, qualified assessment of that person. What you find is that our HCAs are very skilled and very knowledgeable but they haven't had their training and so we are missing out on something vitally important, needing to improve patient care and patient outcomes. We spent three years at university to sit in an office and fill out forms? We are in danger of losing that time to care.

Ben talks openly about how he copes at work. We can see how he has adopted several strategies to help him and his colleagues cope better 'in the line of fire'. He has been able to identify and hold on to the values that he came into nursing with and discusses how he manages to remind himself of these. Using mindfulness techniques appears to help with self-care – he is demonstrating compassion towards himself.

Importantly, Ben talks about how he tries to maintain his values at difficult times and uses the process of reflection and feedback to do this. Staff are also encouraged to reflect in and on action (Schön, 1983), as described in Chapter 7, in order to make sure that they are demonstrating the values that they want to demonstrate. Ben works hard to maintain the boundaries of the nursing profession and is courageous in speaking out on behalf of the team if he feels that they are being asked to do tasks that are not in the nursing remit. As well as working to his own values, he is also using the prescribed values of the NMC Code (NMC, 2015):

- Prioritise people
- Practise effectively
- Preserve safety
- Promote professionalism

Ben also discusses how he works with his team in order to encourage individual and team supportive reflective practice so as to encourage value-checking and values-based practice.

Conclusion

This chapter has hopefully helped you to explore why you came into nursing and also what values keep you in nursing. We have looked at what we mean by 'values' and the challenges of working within a set of prescribed values in a culturally diverse organisation. We have touched upon the notion of the 'wounded healer', which may or may not be a driving force in your choice of career. Whilst this notion of vulnerability may hold up a challenging mirror to us, it can be a useful concept to explore so as to help us 'heal', it can also help us reduce our anxieties and connect with patients in a more compassionate way, which can only benefit the creation of therapeutic relationships with our patients.

Ballatt and Campling encourage us, when working with colleagues and patients, to apply intelligent kindness and adopt an attitude and philosophy that 'unsentimentally values kinship and kindness, understanding their creative, motivating power' (2014: 175). Creating time and space to explore a reconnection with personal and team values can lead to a shared and more consistent base of what we 'do' as nurses and what our professional boundaries are. We then have a stronger voice to use in order to challenge what we feel to be a dissonance between being caught in the dilemma of knowing what is right for our patients and ourselves when having to make difficult and complex clinical decisions.

References

Ballatt, J. and Campling, P. (2014) *Intelligent Kindness: Reforming the Culture of Healthcare*. London: Royal College of Psychiatrists.

Butterworth T. and Shaw T. (2017) *Playing Our Part; The Work Of Graduate And Registered Mental Health Nurses*. London: The Foundation of Nursing Studies. ISBN 978-0-9955785-0-0.

Cummings, J. and Bennett, V. (2012) *Compassion in Practice: Nursing, Midwifery and Care Staff: Our Vision and Strategy*. Leeds: Department of Health.

Department of Health (DH) (2006) *From Values to Action: The Chief Nursing Officer's Review of Mental Health Nursing*. London: DH.

Dinmohammadi, M., Peyrovi, H. and Mehrdad, N. (2013) 'Concept analysis of professional socialization in nursing', *Nursing Forum*, 48: 26–34.

Francis, R. (2013) *Report of the Mid Staffordshire NHS Foundation Trust Public Inquiry, Vol. 1: Analysis of Evidence and Lessons Learned (Part 1)*, HC 898-I. London: The Stationery Office. Available at: http://webarchive.nationalarchives.gov.uk/20150407084003/www.midstaffs publicinquiry.com/sites/default/files/report/Volume%201.pdf (accessed 10 March 2017).

Fulford, K.W.M. (2004) 'Ten principles of values-based medicine', in J. Radden (ed.), *The Philosophy of Psychiatry: A Companion*. New York: Oxford University Press.

Gilbert, P. and Stickley, T. (2012) 'Wounded healers: The role of lived-experience in mental health education and practice', *Journal of Mental Health Education and Practice*, 7 (1): 33–41.

Holt, J. (2017) 'Professional issues', in D. Sellman and P. Snelling (eds), *Becoming a Nurse: Fundamentals of Professional Practice for Nursing*. Abingdon: Routledge.

Jung, C.G. (1977) *The Collected Works of C.G. Jung*, original from University of Minnesota. New York: Pantheon Books.

McClendon, P. (2005) 'Discovery of connections – Societal needs, nursing practice, and caring-healing theory: My story', *International Journal for Human Caring*, 9 (4): 8–13.

NHS (2015) *NHS Constitution*. Available at: www.gov.uk/government/uploads/system/uploads/attachment_data/file/480482/NHS_Constitution_WEB.pdf (accessed 1 October 2017).

Niven, E. (2008) 'The wounded healer: What has the concept to offer nursing?', *Nursing Ethics*, 15 (3): 287–8.

Nursing and Midwifery Council (NMC) (2015) *The Code: Professional Standards of Practice and Behaviour for Nurses and Midwives*. London: NMC.

Pattison, S. and Thomas, B. (2010) 'Healthcare professions and their changing values: Pulling professions together', in S. Pattison, B. Hannigan, R. Pill and B. Thomas (eds), *Emerging Values in Healthcare*. London: Jessica Kingsley Publishers.

Price, S.L. (2009) 'Becoming a nurse: A meta-study of early professional socialization and career choice in nursing', *Journal of Advanced Nursing*, 65 (1): 11–19.

Schön, D.A. (1983) *The Reflective Practitioner*. London: Temple Smith.

Sedgwick, D. (1994) *The Wounded Healer: Countertransference from a Jungian Perspective*. London: Routledge.

Sellman, D. (2011) *What Makes a Good Nurse*. London: Jessica Kingsley Publishing.

Sellman, D. and Snelling, P. (2017) *Becoming a Nurse: Fundamentals of Professional Practice for Nursing*. Abingdon: Routledge.

Stacey, G., Johnson, K., Stickley, T. and Diamond, B. (2011) 'How do nurses cope when values and practice conflict?', *Nursing Times*, 107 (5): 20–23.

Traynor, M. and Buus, N. (2016) 'Professional identity in nursing: UK students' explanation for poor standards of care', *Social Science and Medicine*, 166: 186–94.

Watson, J. (1988) 'New dimensions of human caring theory', *Nursing Science Quarterly*, 1 (4): 175–81.

Watson, J. (2001) 'Theory in human caring', in M. Parker (ed.), *Nursing Theories and Nursing Practice*. Philadelphia, PA: F.A. Davis.

Watson, R. (2012) 'So you think you can care', in W. McSherry, R. McSherry and R. Watson (eds), *Care in Nursing: Principles, Values and Skills*. New York: Oxford University Press.

Woodbridge, K. and Fulford, B. (2005) *Whose Values? A Workbook for Values-Based Practice in Mental Health Care*. London: Sainsbury Centre for Mental Health.

Nursing and Mindfulness
Caroline Barratt and Tess Wagstaffe

We have a finite amount of energy to spend every day before becoming
exhausted. Mindfulness helps you use your energy wisely, spending it on
situations, people and causes that bring you the most joy, meaning and peace.
(Hanh and Cheung, 2011: 7)

Chapter aims

- Introduce mindfulness.
- Discuss how mindfulness can benefit nurses.
- Understand how nurses have integrated mindfulness into their professional practice through case studies.
- Develop mindfulness techniques.
- Explore common questions about mindfulness.

Introduction

The inclusion of a chapter on mindfulness practice in this book for nurses reflects the personal experiences of the authors of the benefits of mindfulness practice, in both their professional and personal lives, as well as reflecting a growing evidence base that suggest the potential of mindfulness to improve the well-being of health professionals. However, it is not just about using mindfulness practice to cope with difficulty. We also explore the potential of mindfulness to help us build relationships, with ourselves, patients and colleagues; support the creation of positive working environments; improve patient safety; and putting nurses back in touch with why they engage in the work they do and the joy therein.

This chapter includes some activities that you may wish to engage in. Mindfulness doesn't really mean anything while it remains an abstract or intellectual concept. It is something that needs to be experienced. Please take care of yourself throughout your exploration of mindfulness. It is possible to experience strong and difficult emotions as well as calmness and positive states of mind, so it is important to take into account your current state of mind and capacity for engaging in these exercises. If you do experience difficulties or feel uncertain, we would recommend stopping any further mindfulness practices and seeking the guidance of an experienced mindfulness teacher.

What is Mindfulness?

Interest in mindfulness training to support the well-being and professional practice of health professionals has grown significantly in the last 20 years. The evidence about how mindfulness practice can impact health professionals suggests that the development of mindfulness can help to protect healthcare professionals, including students, from burnout and stress (Burton et al., 2016; Craigie et al., 2016; Horner et al., 2014; Shapiro et al., 2005; Gockel et al., 2013; Newsome et al., 2012; Gauthier et al., 2015; Cohen-Katz etal., 2005). For students training to be healthcare professionals, mindfulness practice has also been associated with improved patient care (Shapiro et al., 1998; Shields, 2011; Warnecke et al., 2011). A critical interpretative synthesis of findings from qualitative research on the impact of mindfulness training on nurses and midwives concluded that mindfulness created a:

> quiet mental space giving them agency and perspective and leading to improved caring, including a more patient-centred focus and increased presence and listening. Mindfulness appears to alter the way nurses and midwives operate within a stressful work environment, thereby changing the way the environment is experienced by themselves and, potentially, the people in their care. (Hunter, 2016: 918)

Other nursing literature, such as Watson's Human Caring Theory (Sitzman and Watson, 2013) and Parse's concept of 'true presence' (Palmieri and Kiteley, 2012), has also drawn on the concept of mindfulness as a mechanism of improving connection and quality of care.

There is, however, some criticism of the evidence base for the effectiveness of mindfulness, particularly due to methodological issues such small sample sizes, lack of control groups and failure to investigate side effects, which means that the benefits of mindfulness may have been overemphasised and the risks overlooked (Farias and Wikholm, 2016; Lomas et al., 2015).

What it means to be 'mindful' or 'practice mindfulness' is currently a matter of much debate. The complex historical and spiritual roots of the term in Buddhist philosophy and the variety of definitions for 'mindfulness' make its translation in

Westernised mindfulness teaching difficult (Stanley, 2013). Kabat-Zinn is often credited with the initial work in which the concept of mindfulness was integrated into a training course to improve well-being at the University of Massachusetts Medical School. That course is now known as Mindfulness-Based Stress Reduction (MBSR). Kabat-Zinn defines mindfulness as: 'paying attention in a particular way; on purpose, in the present moment, and non-judgmentally' (1994: 4). We can therefore start thinking about mindfulness as getting out of 'autopilot', dominated by constant thoughts and judgements, and become more aware and present in our moment-to-moment experience. Kabat Zinn describes the reason for doing this:

> when you begin paying attention to what your mind is doing, you will probably find that there is a great deal of mental and emotional activity going on beneath the surface. These incessant thoughts and feelings can drain a lot of your energy. They can be obstacles to experiencing even brief moments of stillness and contentment. (2004: 25)

Our minds are rarely still. Not only are we thinking about what we are doing at the time but we are also thinking about what happened that morning, the argument we just had with a colleague or what we will make for dinner in the evening. Not only does our busy mind create suffering but it also prevents us from noticing and being present within the joyful and happy moments in life. This quote from Hanh helps to convey what is meant by 'being mindful' during a particular activity and how it can alter the experience of being alive. Here, he focuses on washing-up:

> If while washing dishes, we think only of the cup of tea that awaits us, thus hurrying to get the dishes out of the way as if they were a nuisance, then we are not 'washing the dishes to wash the dishes'. What's more, we are not alive during the time we are washing the dishes. In fact we are completely incapable of realising the miracle of life while standing at the sink. If we can't wash the dishes, the chances are we won't be able to drink our tea either. While drinking the cup of tea, we will only be thinking of other things, barely aware of the cup in our hands. Thus we are sucked away into the future and we are incapable of actually living one minute of life. (1987: 4)

In terms of nursing practice, when we are attending to a person's personal care or assessing a person's mental or physical health whilst being preoccupied with an endless list of other tasks, we may not only be missing out on gathering information, listening attentively or focusing on the task in hand, but we are also at risk of missing out on moments of connectedness with our patients. These are moments in which we can perhaps reconnect with why we do what we do and, in turn, find satisfaction and pleasure within our role as a nurse.

Therefore, developing mindfulness is not just about becoming more present in and aware of our suffering, it has the potential to wake us up in all aspects of our lives and thankfully that includes moments of joy, love and connection in both our work and personal lives.

Activity 5.1   The Pause

A first step in developing mindfulness is learning to stop and notice our current experience. It can be useful to regularly take a pause in our daily life as a way of learning to check in and notice how we are. This exercise can be used as many times as you would like throughout the day:

1.   Stop what you are doing. You can remain seated or standing.
2.   If appropriate for where you are, you can close your eyes.
3.   Bring your attention to your breathing and follow the breath cycle for 10–15 breaths. There is no need to breathe deeply or in any particular way.
4.   When you are ready, open your eyes.

Try this at different times during the day. How does it affect you?

Writing from a Buddhist perspective, Subhuti describes that, in general, the term *mindfulness* 'may refer either to a particular quality of consciousness or to the effort to create that quality of consciousness in oneself … But, whether we are thinking of the product or the process, mindfulness clearly has to do with the highest possible lucidity and clarity of mind' (2015: 190). He describes how Buddhist discourse emphasises three aspects of mindfulness: attentiveness, awareness and vigilance. Subhuti describes 'attentiveness' as becoming more aware of sensory experience – the direct experience of a given moment as opposed to being caught up in a mental dialogue about it. The ability to attend to experience in this way can be developed through training the mind in the ability to focus and concentrate. Modern definitions of mindfulness, such as Kabat-Zinn's described in the introduction, tend to focus on the attentiveness aspect of mindfulness.

However, attentiveness to experience practiced in isolation may lead to a practice in which the practitioner is detached from the context in which the experience is arising. Without a broader 'awareness', there is a lack of clarity about where we are, our motivations for doing what we are doing and why we are participating in that activity. This is important for you as a nurse, for whom becoming narrowly focused and losing a sense of the wider context is clearly potentially problematic for patient care. Developing awareness supports our attentiveness by supporting a broader sense of what is going on within our experience and how it relates to others. In caring for others, this is particularly important. It is important that we are attentive to our own sensory experience but without a broader awareness – which also acknowledges the experience of the person we are caring for within the context around us – we will not be effective.

Lastly, Subhuti (2015) refers to the importance of 'vigilance', which he describes as the ethical quality that is informing our actions and state of mind. Is the way in which we are behaving or thinking indicative of kindness and compassion, the values that we wish to model? Or has a more negative mental state crept in to cause us to act in ways that don't align to the values that we hold?

So, mindfulness is not necessarily just about 'bare attention' and non-judgement in the present moment. That is a very good place for us to start in terms of developing our mindfulness practice but, in itself, it only presents part of the picture. Whilst your own experience of caring for another is important, clearly it is important to hold that within a broader awareness of the situation and the needs of your patients and colleagues, you must not become isolated or disconnected from them.

∙∙

Activity 5.2   Becoming Aware of Distraction

To be more present, it can be helpful to develop awareness of how distracted we often are and so this is the focus of this second activity.

When caring for patients, start to become aware of where your attention is and to what extent you are 'present' with the person you are caring for. At the end of your shift, note down what distracts you and pulls your attention away from providing care. You may wish to consider:

- Sensory experience, such as smells, sounds, pain and hunger.
- Emotions, such as emotions arising that make it difficult to focus and be present.
- Thoughts, such as mental chatter about issues that you are not immediately concerned with, planning for what is next or judgements about the situation.

You may find it useful to ask a colleague to do the activity, too, so that you can then discuss what you notice and explore the implications for practice.

Source: Adapted from Barratt (2017)

∙∙

Attitudinal Foundations of Mindfulness and their Role in Nursing

Another way to explore mindfulness is to consider what Kabat-Zinn refers to as the 'Seven Attitudinal Foundations' (2004) (Figure 5.1). These foundations describe the qualities that are helpful in the cultivation of mindful awareness.

Beginner's mind – In order to become more present, we need to start to become aware of the assumptions and beliefs that prevent us from seeing things as they are. 'Beginner's mind' is the willingness to see things as though we have not seen them before. It is the cultivation of curiosity and interest even in situations that are familiar to us, so that we are attentive to what is happening rather than relying on mental constructions of what we think is happening based on previous experience. Whilst as nurses we are aware of the importance of our knowledge of previous health history, or perhaps previous risk assessments, it is important to combine this with paying attention to the situation as it presents itself at the time. Brandon explained

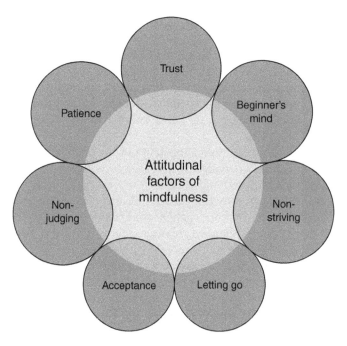

Figure 5.1 Seven attitudinal foundations of mindfulness (adapted from Kabat-Zinn, 2004)

how there are times when our minds are 'wandering so much that here no room for anything that is being said. One is just there physically' (Brandon, 1990: 6), and assumptions can lead us almost to make decisions before we have completed the new assessment and risk, missing new signs or symptoms. Developing a beginner's mind can help overcome these risks.

Non-striving – In everyday life, we engage in tasks with the hope of seeing a particular outcome. We administer medication with the hope of making patients better, we sit and talk with a patient in the hope that they will feel brighter, or comforted or engage a patient in therapy in the hope that their depressed mood will change or they will stop self-harming. However, in developing mindfulness, this attitude is not helpful as it suggests that in order for things to be 'ok', something needs to happen, something needs to change. This thought prevents us from being present with whatever it is that is happening. For nurses, a perceived lack of therapeutic success can lead to feelings of frustration, burnout and disengagement from our patients. This can also prevent us from engaging or recognising the positive contributions that we make to patient care that do not result in a 'cure' or an outcome that we judge to be successful. Rogers asserts that when we are open to different outcomes, we can 'realize the vital strength of the capacity and potentiality of the individual for constructive action' (Rogers, 1951: 48).

Letting go – As we become more mindful and more sensitive to our thoughts and feelings, we may find that there are thoughts, beliefs or feelings that we cling to.

Wanting things to be a certain way or wanting other people to act in particular ways can be a cause of tension and stress. Mindfulness practices ask that we are open to however things are and to do what we need to do in order to let go. Whilst at work, it can be easy to get caught up in a general sense of stress in the workplace or to start ruminating on an issue with a colleague or patient. By bringing ourselves into the present moment, we are more able to let this go and focus on what is in front of us rather than clinging to thoughts about the way something should or shouldn't be.

Acceptance – When difficult things happen in our life or at work, for example the death of a patient, we make a clinical error or disagree with a colleague, and we tend to go through a process of denial and anger before starting to develop some level of acceptance. Arguing with the way things are is ultimately fruitless and can prolong our suffering. Very often, we cannot change what has happened and, if there is the possibility of changing things, then we are often unable to see it until we can accept what is going on and work with it in a more creative way.

Non-judging – Intrinsic to the development of mindfulness is becoming aware of the constant stream of judgement that our minds engage in and becoming able to stand back from that. The ability to do this means that we are not caught up in our mental judgements about the situation we are in. This increases the possibility of being present in our experience and responding appropriately to it rather than reacting based on unconscious habits that have developed in response to our judgements. Within nursing, we are constantly required to think critically and continuously reflect on our practice, which has the potential to manifest itself in being judgemental towards ourselves in a negative and unhelpful way that can greatly impact on our well-being. This will be explored further in Chapter 7, titled 'Self compassion'. We may also engage in judgement of others, which can often colour our interactions with them, causing us to label them as 'problematic' even before we have greeted them on that occasion.

Patience – Kabat-Zinn describes patience as a 'form of wisdom', the cultivation of which shows that we 'accept that the fact that sometimes things must unfold in their own time' (2004: 34). As we become more aware of our minds and bodies and the suffering we can experience in relation to them, learning to hold that with gentleness and patience is important. Patience gives us the room to allow what is there to be there and not to be in a hurry to change it or ourselves in a forced, strident way. Trying to integrate mindfulness into nursing practice is a challenge, so we need to ensure that we are patient with ourselves as we try to develop new ways of working and being.

Trust – As we become more present and aware, we become more able to listen to our feelings and intuition. This enables us to identify the most skilful responses to the situations in which we find ourselves and we start to trust ourselves more and more. We start to notice the judgements and assumptions of others and are less blown about by those with strong opinions, and with awareness we are able to bring ourselves back to our experience and use that as the basis for our decision-making. This is likely to influence our self-confidence as a nurse and, paradoxically, as we start to trust ourselves more, and become less defensive, being open to the views of others becomes less threatening.

Developing mindfulness

There are many ways to develop mindfulness and it is important that you don't feel forced to engage in any one particular practice, but explore what suits you. Mindfulness practices fall into two rough groups: formal and informal.

'Formal practices' are those that require you to take time out from your normal activities to engage in them. This may include meditation practices such as the Breath Awareness Practice, which involves focusing on the breath usually whilst seated and with the eyes closed; or Body Scan, which involves focusing on different parts of the body in a sequential process, this is usually done lying down with the eyes closed. The time taken can vary considerably from five minutes to an hour.

'Informal practices', such as 'The Pause' in Activity 5.1 or 'Becoming aware of distraction' in Activity 5.2 can be done within your everyday life, providing an opportunity to become aware and present within the flow of the day. The most effective way of developing mindfulness is by combining formal and informal practices and engaging in them regularly. Reading about mindfulness is not sufficient. Conceptual and experiential understanding are not the same, so engaging in practice is an important element of coming to appreciate what is meant by 'mindfulness'.

There are now many resources on mindfulness available online as well as in books. The References section at the end of the chapter includes some helpful resources in this regard. However, we have found that engaging with an experienced mindfulness teacher who has a committed mindfulness practice themselves can be very valuable in developing a mindfulness practice. Opportunities for training are often available in the workplace and, if you are not aware of any it, may be worth enquiring. You may also wish to consider taking a course such as Mindfulness-Based Stress Reduction (MBSR), which gives an experiential introduction to mindfulness.

Although mindfulness meditation is usually well tolerated, it has been associated with side effects such as anxiety and psychosis (Farias and Wikholm, 2016) and, as yet, insufficient research has been carried out to establish why this is the case or who is particularly at risk (Dobkin et al., 2012). We have chosen the exercises and suggestions in this chapter with your safety and well-being in mind, avoiding extended periods of meditation, but be attentive to your own needs and limits. If you have suffered from recent trauma, bereavement or are suffering an acute period of mental illness, then be cautious, particularly around periods of silent mindfulness meditation, and seek out an experienced and suitably qualified mindfulness teacher if, after having read this chapter, you wish to explore things in more depth.

Mindfulness, nursing and resilience

Hopefully, from the discussion of what mindfulness is, you are starting to get a sense of why mindfulness is relevant to you. However, we now move on to draw out some of the most salient points about why mindfulness practice may be particularly useful for nurses. We provide specific examples so that you can start to explore in your own mind and experience the relevance to your professional practice.

Noticing Thoughts and How They Impact Experience

> I'm not saying that thinking is bad. Like everything else, it's useful in moderation. A good servant, but a bad master. (Watts, 2013)

As we have already said, the aim of mindfulness is not to stop thinking. Thinking is a useful tool— 'a good servant', as Watts suggests above. As nurses, the wealth of knowledge that you have built up through your training and experience is not forgotten or put aside during mindful nursing practice. Thought is an essential tool in your decision-making, a way of drawing on the knowledge that you have.

However, mindfulness can help us change our relationship to thought. It is possible for us to get stuck in unhelpful cycles of thought about our experience that can make us feel worse and prevent us from seeing what is going on. It is also possible for our underlying beliefs and assumptions to affect how we perceive our experience and influence how we react in any given situation. Becoming aware of what is influencing our perception allows us to step to one side and take a fresh look. Developing mindfulness means that we develop the ability to be less caught up in the mental dialogues about what is going on in our lives, and the wrong or right of it, and become better able to identify what our actual experience of it is. This does not mean that mindfulness practice will instantly make us feel better, or that difficult emotions will never affect us, but it does mean that we can have greater insight and increase the possibility that we can intervene and not get trapped in unconscious patterns of thoughts that cause us distress.

Thinking, stress and suffering

As we have already discussed, our minds tend to jump around from thought to thought, but our minds can also get stuck on a particular thought pattern that might be unhelpful. For example, when I am tired and feeling overwhelmed at work, I only notice tasks that I feel I could have completed better, or remember conversations with patients or relatives that I feel did not go as well as I would have liked. I have noticed that it is this thought pattern and this constant anticipation of feeling overwhelmed that is causing much of the stress and poor confidence.

Even when I sit down to relax, I feel stressed and anxious because my mind is still caught up. This can also happen when I get in from work and I continue to ruminate over how I could have performed better, within my role, or how difficult it feels at times. This means that the anxiety gets prolonged and eats into the apparently relaxing and pleasant aspects of our lives.

. . . .

Activity 5.3   Identifying negative thoughts

Identifying what negative thoughts and stories our mind gets stuck on can be very helpful and is the focus of this activity. If, however, you find the task upsetting or that the focus makes you more stressed, perhaps you can try the activity at a different time with the support of a friend or colleague. Make sure that you take care of yourself.

Over the next week, pay attention to stressful or difficult thoughts or trains of thought that get repeated in your mind even when you have no wish to think about those issues. You may wish to make a note of:

1.   What are these thoughts about? For example, work, family, money, etc.?
2.   When are these thoughts most prevalent?
3.   What is your experience of your physical body whilst thinking about it? For example, is there pain or tension in the body? How is your heart rate and breathing?
4.   What emotions are present?
5.   What effect does bringing awareness to these thoughts have on your experience of them?

. . . .

Through mindfulness practice, we can become aware of the things that pull us away from where we actually want our mind to be. Often, these distractions are fuelled by our fear of suffering. This includes the whole spectrum of human difficulties, from the small frustrations of writing to the painful experiences of illness and grief. Thomas Merton wrote:

> The more you try to avoid suffering, the more you suffer, because smaller and more insignificant things begin to torture you, in proportion to your fear of being hurt. The one who does most to avoid suffering is, in the end, the one who suffers most. (1948: 91)

Nurses are constantly exposed to the most challenging aspects of human life – those events that cause the most pain and suffering. It is not surprising then that nurses often experience stress and burnout. Being able to recognise that we are in pain or experiencing difficulty and being able to then respond appropriately is fundamental in self-care and is something that can arise through the development of mindfulness. This will also be explored in Chapter 7.

Using mindfulness in our working with others

Central to the idea of mindfulness is the idea of being present, aware and open to our present moment experience. In particular, this relates to developing our ability to control where we place our attention, to become less vulnerable to our 'monkey minds' and take ourselves out of 'autopilot mode', which can dominate our lives. Halifax (2014) developed the GRACE model of interacting with patients that encourages a mindful approach by helping to focus our intention as we first step into a relationship with the patient, encouraging meaningful and helpful interaction and then bringing the encounter to an end. Halifax describes how the GRACE model can support compassionate care:

> Clinicians often do not take a 'reflective pause' but jump into immediately assessing the patient before getting attentionally and ethically grounded, seeing their biases, then sensing into the patient's experience before making a clinical assessment. The GRACE process can guide a nurse into that moment (or moments) of reflection that can provide the base for healthy, grounded and principled compassion. (Ibid.: 123)

The stages of the GRACE model are shown in Figure 5.2 and are discussed below. In the *first stage* of gathering attention, Halifax suggests that we take just a moment to notice where our attention is, perhaps becoming aware of the in-breath or sense of feet on the floor to help us become present.

In the *second stage*, she suggests we bring to mind our intention, get in touch with a sense of why we are about to engage with that person and the values that we seek to embody while doing it. We do not often think about the values that bring us to the work that we do and, yet, for many nurses, it was a strong sense of vocation and a desire to care that brought them into the profession. Bringing this to mind during the workday may be a source of support for us as it helps reconnect us to our sense of purpose, which is often lost in the busyness of everyday healthcare delivery. It should be noted that neither of these stages needs to take any more than a few

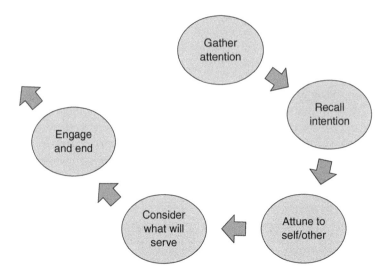

Figure 5.2   GRACE model of compassion care (adapted from Halifax, 2014: 123)

seconds – Halifax is not suggesting that we take a break every time we move on to a new person!

In the *third stage*, we attune first to ourselves, how we are feeling, the thoughts that are arising as we start to move towards engaging with this person. Having become aware of these, we become more conscious of what we are bringing with us into the interaction and how what we are feeling and experiencing might affect our perception of the person for whom we are caring. Then, we attune to the other person, having noticed our own biases and subjectivity and using that as the basis for empathy, we orientate our attention to the other person.

In the *fourth stage*, we consider what will serve, explicitly bringing to mind relevant experience and knowledge that is relevant to identify what needs to be done. Halifax described how this process of discernment 'requires attentional and affective balance, a deep sense of moral grounding and an ethical imperative, as well as an unbiased attunement into the patient's experience and needs' (2014: 124), which is what is established in the first three stages of the model.

In *fifth stage*, we engage with the patient, carrying out the work that needs to be done before finding a way to end the encounter. Halifax places strong emphasis on setting up before engaging with the patient by first getting in touch with yourself, becoming aware and present. Equally, she then emphasises the importance of needing to consciously end the interaction, to: 'acknowledge internally and often interpersonally what has transpired'. Failure to do this may make it difficult to move on to the next task because, mentally, you may remain caught up in previous encounters that, although no longer actually happening, remain live either emotionally or in our thoughts or both.

It is important to note that although we have discussed this model in relation to working with patients, it is equally applicable in any encounter that we have. Its value is particularly powerful in interactions that may be problematic such as with a difficult colleague or manager. Grounding ourselves before engaging, especially at times where we feel an emotional charge or particularly vulnerable, can help to create space for skilful responses as opposed to reactions based on habit.

Finding the joy: Becoming mindful of what we give and what we receive

As we said earlier, becoming mindful is not just about recognising the difficult or challenging aspects of our lives. We can also become more aware of moments of joy, happiness and beauty, more able to feel them deeply and become better at noticing them within our own experience. In a qualitative study of the impact of mindfulness training on nurses by Cohen-Katz et al. (2005: 84), they cited a nurse who had been on an MBSR course, which includes a task in which they are asked to observe and record pleasant events over the week, like saying:

> When looking for a pleasant event, I kept looking for something really big. Then I realised that the simple interactions with others in my life are the ones that are the most pleasurable – really noticing how it feels when my husband's arms are around me in bed or hugging my child and stroking her hair ...

We can train ourselves to start to notice pleasant experiences when they arise but this is challenging if we have become used to living in states of stress and anxiety. The phenomenon of confirmation bias describes how people pay more attention, and give more weight, to information that confirms their current position or beliefs (Wason, 1960). Whilst a little oversimplistic, an example of this is if we have decided that, today, 'I got out of the wrong side of bed,' we will naturally be drawn to noticing the aspects of our experience that confirm this – the person who pulls out on us on the motor way; the negative comment from a colleague; the milk running out – as opposed to those aspects of your experience that may present a different case: your partner making you a cup of tea; the flowers in your front garden; the person who let you out at that busy junction. This is not to say that there aren't difficult circumstances in our lives and jobs that are demanding and draining but, as we learn to pay attention, we start to notice the variability of our experience and the aspects of our experience that don't fit with our dominant narratives.

This is just one very particular example about a given day but imagine these patterns writ large over the whole course of our lives? How much are we missing? In order to work that out, we have to stop and notice – which is the first step in mindfulness practice. Activity 5.4 provides a way of starting to reconnect with the positive aspects of our experience.

Activity 5.4   Shifting Our Focus to Change Our Experience

Where we choose to place our attention has a huge impact on how we experience the world. As human beings, we are wired to notice threat and, as such, tend to focus on negative experiences. Have you noticed how despite all the people you might help in one day, all of them will be forgotten as you focus on the one person whom you couldn't help or the mistake that you made?

This task has two elements. At the end of each day, sit down and write:

1.   At least three things that you have done to help others, where you are able to appreciate the contribution that you made to their lives (personally or professionally).

They do not have to be big things! Making someone a cup of tea, giving your time to chat with a friend, holding a patient's hand to ease their fear, remembering to say 'Happy Birthday!' to a colleague ... these are worthy of recognition and celebration.

2.   At least three things that you are grateful for that day.

Again, they do not have to be big things! Perhaps seeing the sunshine as you walked from your car into work, a patient who said 'Thank you,' a nice meal.

These are exercises that help to retune our attention so that we start to become increasingly conscious of the positive aspects of our lives.

Nursing and Mindfulness: Frequently Asked Questions

In this section, we take three key questions that are often raised about mindfulness and nursing as a way of exploring how mindfulness is relevant to nurses and within nursing practice:

1. At times, when I am feeling really stressed and anxious, I find the mindfulness meditation exercises difficult as the 'space' becomes filled with worry and pre-occupation. I have at times tried the practice before work but, due to the worry, this has been difficult. What would you recommend?

This is a very common experience even amongst experienced mindfulness practitioners. First, it is important to note that the practice of mindfulness meditation does not require us to stop thinking, have a 'clear mind' or be relaxed. This is a common unhelpful misconception. During meditation, the practice is simply to be aware of what is – including the thoughts that arise and fade out during practice as well as the tension that may be present in our bodies. Striving to become calmer or to stop thinking is likely to make the practice more difficult, as you may get more tense when you notice that your experience is not as you wish it to be (you may find it helpful to reread the 'Attitudinal Foundations of Mindfulness and Their Role in Nursing' section above). For example, when engaging in a breath awareness practice, which involves focusing on the experience of the breath, when you realise that you have become distracted from the breath, then you repeatedly bring your attention back to the breath as best you can. Sometimes, it may feel like you do this hundreds of times a minute! Or, perhaps, if you have one dominant story running through your mind, you may completely forget the practice for many minutes at a time. But this does not mean that you are 'bad at mindfulness' or 'can't meditate', it is simply how the practice is today. So, even when we feel like the practice is 'going badly', the invitation is to keep practicing with gentleness, patience and a beginner's mind. Your experience of the practice can change dramatically even within a short time.

Having said this, however, I appreciate how challenging it can be to meditate when your mind is all over the place and I have at times cut meditations short for this reason. When starting out, be realistic about how long you want the mindfulness practice to last. You may find it easier to build up to longer periods of time. Be conscious of what is going on in your life and be kind to yourself regarding whether to engage in a practice, whilst also noticing our tendency to be lazy or put things off. When things are particularly stressful in our lives is when mindfulness becomes most beneficial, yet it can also be the time when practice is the most challenging. Continuing to practice regularly when things are relatively calm is a good way of developing our skills and confidence when conditions are more supportive of our practice:

2. I feel that being hyper-vigilant and forever on alert is an essential part of my role and I am not sure how I can be mindful or in the moment when it is important that I am accountable and responsible for the health and safety of all of my patients.

It is possible to be mindful in any situation that we find ourselves in and being mindful does not mean that we are not able to meet our responsibilities or that we forget everything. It is not about shutting our minds down or disconnecting from what's going on. However, as we become more mindful, there may be a shift in how we relate to the pressure placed on us. When we consciously bring awareness to where we are and what is going on and stop being so caught up in our thoughts about what's going on, which may well be adding to our sense of anxiety, we may deal more effectively with what is in front of us.

Imagine that you have to carry out a procedure with a patient and you know that you are pushed for time, constantly ruminating on thoughts such as 'I must finish this soon as I need to write up those notes and speak to that colleague,' 'I don't have enough time to do this properly,' 'I am not good at doing this,' 'What if I get it wrong?' will not mean that you are more likely to do the procedure well. Constantly thinking about the mistakes that we fear we might make does not protect us from making them – it actually draws our attention away from where it needs to be, on the patient, and it also fuels a negative thought cycle which may contribute to decreased confidence and burnout. Another important aspect is that if we are present, we are better able to identify creative solutions to the issues that cause stress and we become better able to identify and meet our own needs. This may include looking after ourselves better as well as identifying steps to reduce stress in the workplace. It may, of course, also include leaving a job role that becomes too overwhelming for us.

However, we don't expect you to blindly believe us. It is important that if you are curious about the benefits of mindfulness practice that you then find ways of engaging in mindfulness practice – it is not about transforming everything you do overnight but about starting slowly and taking small steps during your day so as to become present and aware.

3. I would like to feel that I can end my day but I often take home my concerns about clinical situations at work or issues with colleagues. I would like to feel that I could leave some of this worry at work. It can feel as though, emotionally, I am on call 24/7 and, sometimes, it is almost a relief to return to work to allay these anxieties.

Earlier in the chapter, we introduced the work of Halifax (2014), who developed the GRACE model of compassionate care-giving. She focuses on endings in recognition of the importance of consciously ending interactions with patients. This can also be applied, and perhaps is even more important, when marking the end of a shift so that you are able to consciously move into other roles in your life and put down the role of being a nurse. Any mindfulness practice aims to develop our capacity to be present, which means that when we are at work, we can be fully present at work, and when we are at home, we can fully engage at home. However, there are particular ways of using mindfulness practice to end your workday:

• When you get into your car at the end of the day, put you key into the ignition and, before you turn it, take several breaths and check in with yourself.

- On the drive home, spend some time without the radio on and be aware of the experience of driving, particularly bring attention to what you are seeing, noticing how this familiar route looks at that time.
- If you use public transport and a phone and headphones, use that time to do a short guided mindfulness practice.
- Place a small notepad in your car or bag so that if anything work-related occurs to you on the way home, you can write it down before arriving home.
- On arriving home, take a pause before entering the house, consciously acknowledging that you are now home and that you can choose to be present here.
- I find it hard to give undivided attention to my patients as I feel that I am always preoccupied with the next 'task' or being aware that there is a job that I have not completed. I like to think or hope that my patients are not aware of my inattention but I am sure that there are times when they are.

Being distracted this way is very common in today's society, which places a lot of value on being busy. That is not to say that your job is not busy! But even within the busyness, we can learn to pay closer attention to what we are doing at any given moment. Sometimes, we might confuse being busy with being efficient but, from my experience, these are not always the same thing. Research suggests that we are actually very poor multitaskers and that mistakes occur due to distraction. Healthcare settings can be chaotic; disruptions and interruptions are significant contributory factors to errors such as drug-administration errors (Kreckler et al., 2008). Perhaps there are times where our perceived hyper-vigilance is an illusion and, in fact, we are in a state of inattention. Practically, we need to consider how to focus and explore ways of ending the previous task before consciously moving our attention to the task in hand (reread the above answer for suggestions on how this might be achieved). It is also important to bear in mind that mindful presence does not need to take up more time and that it may help us to be more efficient and effective, thereby avoiding mistakes and saving time in the long run.

With regards to whether or not patients notice if you are distracted, just consider your own experience for a moment: Can you recall a time when you were trying to talk to someone and they are clearly not engaged with you? It can be quite hurtful and alienating, particularly if we are feeling vulnerable at the time, so it is unlikely that patients are not aware. Furthermore, it is not only the patients who suffer from your lack of presence, it also detracts from your experience as a nurse. Ultimately, you are there to care and, although your role has many different facets, if you are not actually present in those moments of care delivery, you also miss out on the joy and connection that can arise from them which make the work of nursing worthwhile. There are probably not many nurses who would describe writing notes or care plans as one of the more rewarding parts of their role. But, as we said above: when you are writing the notes, be present to writing notes; when you are caring for a patient, be present with the patient; when you are talking with a colleague, talk with a colleague.

When these tasks are interrupted – as they inevitably will be because you are more aware – you can actively choose how to deal with the interruption rather than just reacting. Is it urgent? Does it require your immediate attention? In which case, you choose to shift your attention to the new task. Or can the interruption wait? Be clear with the person who has interrupted you about how much time you need before you can deal with them. Responding in this way means that you don't get pushed and pulled like a bottle on the waves of the sea. However, if you do find yourself getting completely caught up in events, be kind to yourself as you notice this and take a few conscious breaths or feel your feet on the floor as a way of becoming present and reengaging in a more conscious way.

Conclusion

Mindfulness is currently a bit of a buzzword and is often portrayed as something of a cure-all. Although we don't agree with all the 'hype', we do feel that it is useful and, when developed through regular practice, is supportive of nurse well-being as well as effective and compassionate patient care. A last point that we would like to make is that, although much of the discussion in this chapter has been about acceptance and letting go, mindfulness is not about becoming passive or submissive, gallantly coping with whatever is thrown at you. Attention is rightly being drawn to the current stresses in the healthcare working environments and the risks posed by nursing burnout and distress to the quality of care provision and the harm to nurses themselves (see McPherson et al., 2016). Action needs to be taken in order to ensure that the rights of nurses are protected and that working conditions for nurses are improved. However, paradoxically, acceptance of the way things are in the moment can free up energy and facilitate creative action to effect change. Developing a mindfulness practice is therefore not about sticking your head in the sand or being walked all over in the name of 'acceptance' and 'letting go'. It is about being present with what is, both within ourselves and in the world, and then taking action in accordance with our values. Sometimes, this may include advocating for change in the workplace, standing up for a patient or perhaps a career change. But, whatever it is that we do, it is done with awareness, informed by our values and aspirations and not as a knee-jerk reaction, based on old habits and preconceived ideas.

References

Barratt, C. (2017) 'Exploring how mindfulness and self-compassion can enhance compassionate care', *Nursing Standard*, 31 (21): 55–63.

Brandon, D. (1990) *Zen in the Art of Helping*. London: Penguin.

Burton, A., Burgess, C., Dean, S., Koutsopoulou, G.Z. and Hugh-Jones, S. (2016) 'How effective are mindfulness-based interventions for reducing stress among healthcare professionals? A systematic review and meta-analysis', *Stress and Health*, 33 (1): 3–13 (early view).

Cohen-Katz, J., Wiley, S., Capuano, T., Baker, D.M., Deitrick, J. and Shapiro, S. (2005) 'The effects of mindfulness-based stress reduction on nurse stress and burnout: A qualitative and quantitative study, Part III', *Holistic Nursing Practice*, 19 (1): 26–35.

Craigie, M., Slatyer, S., Hegney, D., Osseiran-Moisson, R., Gentry, M., Davis, S., Dolan, T. and Rees, C. (2016) 'A pilot evaluation of a mindful self-care and resiliency (MSCR) intervention for nurses', *Mindfulness*, 7 (3): 764–74.

Dobkin, P.L., Irving, J.A. and Amar, S. (2012) 'For whom may participation in a mindfulness-based stress reduction program be contraindicated?', *Mindfulness*, 3 (1): 44–50. Doi: 10.1007/s12671-011-0079-9.

Farias, M. and Wikholm, C. (2016) 'Has the science of mindfulness lost its mind?', *BJPsych Bulletin*, 40 (6): 329–32. Doi: 10.1192/pb.bp.116.053686.

Gauthier, T., Meyer, R., Grefe, D. and Gold, J. (2015) 'An on-the-job mindfulness-based intervention for pediatric icu nurses: A pilot study', *Journal of Alternative and Complementary Medicine*, 20 (5): A87.

Gockel, A., Cain, T., Malove, S. and James, S. (2013) 'Mindfulness as clinical training: Student perspectives on the utility of mindfulness training in fostering clinical intervention skills', *Journal of Religion & Spirituality in Social Work*, 32 (1): 36–59.

Halifax, J. (2014) 'GRACE for nurses: Cultivating compassion in nurse/patient interactions', *Journal of Nursing Education and Practice*, 4 (1): 121–8. Doi: 10.5430/jnep.v4n1p121.

Hanh, T.N. (1987) *The Miracle of Mindfulness: An Introduction to the Practice of Meditation*. Boston, MA: Beacon Press.

Hanh, T.N. and Cheung, L. (2011) *Mindful Eating, Mindful Life: Savour Every Moment and Every Bite*. New York: HarperCollins.

Horner, J.K., Piercy, B.S., Eure, L. and Woodard, F.K. (2014) 'A pilot study to evaluate mindfulness as a strategy to improve inpatient nurse and patient experiences', *Applied Nursing Research*, 27 (3): 198–201.

Hunter, L. (2016) 'Making time and space: The impact of mindfulness training on nursing and midwifery practice: A critical interpretative synthesis', *Journal of Clinical Nursing*, 25 (7–8): 918–29.

Kabat-Zinn, J. (1994) *Wherever You Go, There You Are: Mindfulness Meditation in Everyday Life*. New York: Hyperion.

Kabat-Zinn, J. (2004) *Full Catastrophe Living: Using the Wisdom of Your Body and Mind to Face Stress, Pain, and Illness*. London: Piatkus.

Kreckler, S., Catchpole, K., Bottomley, M., Handa, A. and McCulloch, P. (2008) 'Interruptions during drug rounds: an observational study', *British Journal of Nursing*, 17 (21): 1326–1330.

Lomas, T., Cartwright, T. Edginton, T. and Ridge, D. (2015) 'A qualitative analysis of experiential challenges associated with meditation practice', *Mindfulness*, 6 (4): 848–60. Doi: 10.1007/s12671-014-0329-8.

McPherson, S., Hiskey, S. and Alderson, Z. (2016) 'Distress in working on dementia wards – A threat to compassionate care: A grounded theory study', *International Journal of Nursing Studies*, 53: 95–104.

Merton, T. (1948) *The Seven Storey Mountain*. Orlando, FL: Harcourt.

Newsome, S., Waldo, M. and Gruszka, C. (2012) 'Mindfulness group work: Preventing stress and increasing self-compassion among helping professionals in training', *Journal for Specialists in Group Work*, 37 (4): 297–311.

Palmieri, G. and Kiteley, C. (2012) 'The gift of true presence: A nursing story where theory and practice meet', *Canadian Oncology Nursing Journal*, 22 (4): 282–6.

Rogers, C.R. (1951) *Client-centered Therapy: Its Current Practice, Implications, and Theory*. Boston, MA: Houghton Mifflin.

Shapiro, S.L., Schwartz, G.E. and Bonner, G. (1998) 'Effects of mindfulness-based stress reduction on medical and premedical students', *Journal of Behavioral Medicine*, 21 (6): 581–99.

Shapiro, S.L., Astin, J.A., Bishop, S.R. and Cordova, M. (2005) 'Mindfulness-based stress reduction for health care professionals: Results from a randomized trial', *International Journal of Stress Management*, 12 (2): 164–76.

Shields, L.R. (2011) 'Teaching mindfulness techniques to nursing students for stress reduction and self-care', PhD thesis, Nursing Practice Systems Change Projects, St. Catherine University, St. Paul, MN. Available at: http://sophia.stkatc.edu/dnp_projects/18/ (accessed 28 January 2014).

Sitzman, K. and Watson, J. (2013) *Caring Science, Mindful Practice: Implementing Watson's Human Caring Theory*. New York: Springer.

Stanley, S. (2013) '"Things said or done long ago are recalled and remembered": The ethics of mindfulness in early Buddhism, psychotherapy and clinical psychology', *European Journal of Psychotherapy & Counselling*, 15 (2): 151–62.

Subhuti (2015) *Mind in Harmony: The Psychology of Buddhist Ethics*. Cambridge: Windhorse Publications.

Warnecke, E., Quinn, S., Ogden, K., Towle, N. and Nelson, M. (2011) 'A randomised controlled trial of the effects of mindfulness practice on medical student stress levels', *Medical Education*, 45 (4): 381–8.

Wason, P.C. (1960) 'On the failure to eliminate hypotheses in a conceptual task', *Quarterly Journal of Experimental Psychology*, 12 (3): 129–40. Doi: 10.1080/17470216008416717.

Watts, A. (2013) *The Art of Meditation*. Available at: www.youtube.com/watch?v=gd2Ot6hLCtM (accessed 12 March 2018).

Thinking, Learning and Working Under Fire

Steve Wood

Chapter aims

- Describe the origins of reflection in nursing and the reasons for which nurses have not widely adopted critical thinking techniques.
- Outline a number of innovative approaches that seek to promote reflective practice in nursing, in a practical, realistic and creative way.

Introduction

In Chapter 2, the personal impact of nursing in contemporary healthcare and the effect of change were considered. Models of reflection have been used since the 1970s as a means of encouraging thoughtful analysis of nursing practice with only modest success. While there have been many positive examples of reflective approaches being adopted – such as the use of clinical supervision in mental health and health coaching in adult nursing – perhaps the problems associated with broader use has been the rigid, structured 'model' approach to promoting and teaching the skills of reflection and the difficulty in then using these models in a busy practice environment. That said, the value of nurses developing their reflective skills akin to Schön's reflective practitioners 'in action' has been shown to correlate with the delivery of high-quality care, evidence-based practice and personal stress reduction.

The Origins of Reflection in Nursing and the Reasons Why Nurses Have Not Widely Adopted Critical Thinking Techniques

What do we mean by 'reflective practice' in nursing?

Boud et al. define 'reflection' as:

> Reflection is an important human activity in which people recapture their experience, think about it, mull over and evaluate it. It is this working with experience that is important in learning. (1985: 43)

Bulman and Schutz describe 'reflective practice' as:

> 'Reviewing experience from practice so that it may be described, analysed, evaluated and consequently used to inform and change future practice. (2013: 6)

Thus, it can be seen that 'reflective practice' can result in critical thinking about one's clinical practice, skills and competency and the practice of other team members, the application of research and evidence-based practice and the delivery of high-quality care. Reflective practice is also concerned with trying to analyse and understand clinical problems that occur or, conversely, evaluating situations that achieved positive care outcomes.

Approaches to reflection can be informal, but it is the more formal models of reflection that have tended to be used within nursing, and specifically pre-registration nursing courses. The importance of reflection is reinforced within these initial education programmes, with students being expected to select and utilise a model of reflection (from the many options) in order to compile portfolios of their learning and skill attainment, use reflective diaries or employ a model for personal reflection within a written assignment. The difficulty with this strategy is that reflection tends to become an enforced approach that is then often not used after the student qualifies as a registered nurse. Nevertheless, continuing learning is a fundamental aspect of professional development and the contribution of reflection to this process is essential.

The models of reflection used in nursing

A basic search engine exploration using a 'model + reflection + nursing' format shows Johns' model of reflection to be the most widely documented framework used within nursing by a considerable margin. This is followed by Gibbs' framework, with Schön's work close behind. Kolb's (1984) reflective cycle is in fourth place, although it is still utilised quite extensively (Table 6.1).

Table 6.1   The models of reflection used in nursing

Model	Returned results
Johns + reflection + nursing	487,000
Gibbs + reflection + nursing	371,000
Schön + reflection + nursing	367,000
Kolb + reflection + nursing	225,000
Driscoll + reflection + nursing	157,000
Boud + reflection + nursing	50,700

Johns' (1995) 'Model of Structured Reflection'

This was initially proffered as a learning theory but has become more widely known as a 'model of reflection'. It uses cue questions to structure and help analyse an experience. This then enables us to break down our experience and reflect on the process and outcome. Johns' (ibid.) work uses Carper's (1978) four patterns of 'knowing' in nursing: empirical, personal, ethical and aesthetic, adding a fifth pattern of 'reflexivity'. This cyclical process follows five stages:

1. *Bringing the mind home*: Creating space for reflection.
2. *Description*: Summarising the incident.
3. *Reflection*: Thinking about the situation and what occurred.
4. *Alternatives*: Generating different ways of interpreting the incident.
5. *Changes*: Summarising the most workable potential solutions.

Johns' model is often utilised for written reflections on nursing practice in portfolios and as a structure for student assignments. The model's popularity seems to stem from the straightforward stages but, while being relatively easy to use, the potential number of suggested questions often has to be reduced so as to ensure that the reflective process is realistic. However, a central concept of the framework ('bringing the mind home') is often overlooked and, yet, it has potentially high relevance to more informal approaches to reflection. This first stage emphasises the importance of generating the 'mental space' for personal learning by creating time for reflection through such techniques as imagery and mindfulness.

Gibbs' (1988) 'Reflective Cycle'

This also evolved as a learning theory but was then utilised in a structured way as a debriefing framework or cycle. It is a frequently used model within pre-registration nursing courses and is often utilised to structure reflection in professional practice and for critical incident analysis. The framework is particularly useful in helping students reflect on the merits of an experience and their learning styles, and so is often considered easier to use than Johns' model. The model uses a similar series of steps:

- *Description*: What happened?
- *Feelings*: What were you thinking and feeling?
- *Evaluation*: What was good and bad about the experience?
- *Analysis*: What sense can you make of the situation?
- *Conclusion*: What else could you have done?
- *Action plan*: If it arose again, what would you do?

Schön's (1983) 'Reflection-in-action'

In Schön's (1983) influential book, *The Reflective Practitioner*, the philosopher comments that practice presents problems that are inherently 'messy, indeterminate situations', which are characterised by 'uncertainty, instability, uniqueness and value conflict' (ibid.: 20). Here, Schön was referring to the process of reflection in professional education, and so his ideas became hugely significant in many professional curricula. He considered experiential learning to be the cornerstone of effective education, and so this may well explain why his work has become so influential in nursing. Schön's approach celebrates the intuitive and artistic styles that can be brought to uncertain situations. These can be seen in the two central components of the model:

- *Reflection-in-action*: Thinking about one's practice while doing it.
- *Reflection-on-action*: Thinking about an experience after the event.

Arguably, it is Schön's concept of 'Reflection-in-action' that is critically relevant to nursing. Schön viewed this as an essential characteristic of 'expert practitioners' who can test out their ideas while directly engaged it an experience: 'Our thinking serves to reshape what we are doing while we are doing it' (1987: 26).

Schön (1987: 13) further describes the process of reflection in action as:

The art of problem framing

Surprise triggers reflection, directed both to the surprising outcome and to the knowing-in-action that led to it. It is as though the performer asked him/herself, what is this? And at the same time, what understandings and strategies of mine have led me to produce this?

The art of improvisation

The performer restructures his/her understanding of the situation-his/her framing of the problem s/he has been trying to solve, his/her picture of what is going on, or the strategy of action he has been employing.

The art of implementation

On the basis of this restructuring, he/she invents a new strategy of action. S/he tries out the new action s/he has invented, running an on-the-spot experiment whose results s/he interprets, in turn, as a 'solution,' an outcome on the whole satisfactory, or else as a new surprise that calls for a new round of reflection and experiment.

(Reproduced with permission of John Wiley and Sons.)

. . . .

Activity 6.1   Examining Professional Practice Using Schön

Identify an example of health-related 'good practice' that you have seen (as a colleague or a patient). This can be anything that you thought was good, well done, impressive, helpful, etc. Thinking about Schön's work, reflect on your 'story' and consider:

- How the person responsible for the 'good practice' identified that there was a problem to be solved (the art of problem framing).
- How he/she tried different approaches to solving the problem (the art of improvisation).
- How he/she put into practice their chosen action that led to the good outcome (the art of implementation).

What common themes developed from your reflection? Do you think that these themes would be the same across all professional groups? Perhaps share your observations with a work colleague?

. . . .

Why nurses do not always use structured reflective techniques in their practice

Given the strong evidence base, it is surprising to note the lack of consistent application of approaches to critical reflection within nursing to date. Why might this be the case? A poll conducted by the author of a group of qualified adult and mental health nurses attending a mentorship seminar elicited the following reasons:

- Reflection has become too formalised.
- Pressure of time owing to the intensity of clinical work.
- The excessive requirements of documenting care events.
- The emotions attached to a situation require quiet reflection rather than a structured approach.
- It is inconvenient to assign time to write up reflections.
- It is preferable to talk and unburden to a colleague.

- Some issues are too personal to document.
- Reflecting in a planned way does not match real-life reflective thinking.
- There is a need to consider individualised approaches to reflection.

The above reasons correlate with the evaluative work undertaken by Barksby et al. (2015), who cite problems with the practical use of staged models and apprehensions regarding who might see the reflective writing. Oelofsen (2012) also underlines the vast number of reflective models available and the need for simplicity of same in practice. While Jasper (2013) explains that, although the techniques to support reflection in nursing are widely known, initiating action needs to become more of a consistent response. Significantly, de Vries and Timmins (2015) claim that ineffective reflective practice can even contribute to poor quality of care. To help counteract this, de Vries and Timmins (ibid.) further call for greater understanding of the impact of the processes associated with reflection such as removing obstacles. Once the barriers have been identified, it then becomes necessary to remove these before reflection can be undertaken (Caldwell and Grobbel, 2013). With this point in mind, the procedure for dealing with barriers as advocated by Boud et al. (1985) is useful:

1. Acknowledge barriers.
2. Name the barriers.
3. Ask how the barriers operate and their origin.
4. Work with the barriers.

··

Activity 6.2   Examining Professional Practice Using Schön (*cont.*)

Consider repeating the poll that I conducted with mentors, with nurses from your clinical team, and then try to think creatively about how you and your clinical team can work on removing these barriers.

··

Innovative Approaches That Seek to Promote Reflective Practice in a Practical, Realistic and Creative Way

Caldwell and Grobbel (2013) conducted a literature review on the importance of reflection in nursing. The outcome of this review identified four themes:

- *Development of practice* – Reflection has the potential to enhance nursing practice.
- *Emotional impact* – Reflection provides a safe opportunity for nurses to explore their feelings and emotions.

- *Mentor support* – With support from mentors, students can partake in expressive reflection.
- *Barriers* – Acknowledging the barriers will assist in making the required changes for reflection in practice.

Thus, it is evident that reflection can help to reduce anxiety or feelings attached to stressful events or challenging situations encountered in clinical situations. With the potential benefits of reflection in mind, the following questions were posed to a group of final-year work-based learning student nurses in a supervision session:

- How and when do you reflect?
- Do you prefer formal or informal techniques?
- What advice would you give to a new nurse about reflection?

Reflective writing, using some of the techniques outlined in this chapter, are built into the work-based learning pre-registration nursing course. The feedback received seemed to demonstrate that reflection was relatively widely used. The emotional labour of nursing was clearly identifiable and the importance of critical thinking as a means of helping to cope with such stressful situations was evident. It was further apparent that a range of methods was utilised with many being informal. Yet, formal methods were also seen as necessary, with reflection being recommended as an essential learning tool. The responses further provided some suggested options for reflection such as note-taking, supervision, group debriefings, reflecting on events, returning to personal reflections, peer reflection and contemplative activities. The requirement for a supportive structure was also mentioned and as was the need for colleagues to give and be receptive to constructive feedback.

Comparable feedback on critical thinking was documented by Tashiro et al. (2013), who conducted a thematic analysis and then described the attributes, antecedents and consequences of reflection in nursing. One of the aims of this review was to help nurses enhance their reflective skills. The authors describe how, through reflection, nurses develop self-awareness that then expands care skills and promotes excellence and professionalism. Communication with service users and team members is also enhanced, and self-directed learning improved.

Similarly, a particularly useful way of dealing with some of the pressures implicit in clinical nursing practice is striving to attain the high level of 'reflection-in-action' embodied in Schön's 'reflective practitioner' framework. Schön's 'excellent practitioner' is perceived by nursing students (as cited to the chapter author) as a nurse who has maintained their enthusiasm and motivation to provide high-quality care and who utilises both structured reflection approaches and 'reflection-in-action'.

With this observation in mind, and given the strong evidence base for the use of reflection in nursing, one way of dealing with the pressure of working in contemporary healthcare could be by using the strengths of models of reflection, self-reflection and reflection-in-action in a more integrated, realistic, usable, creative and practical way. How might such an aim be achieved? The following suggestions outline some options that could be tested by the practitioner in the clinical setting. Many of these are based on ideas put forward by registered adult and mental health nurses and so are currently being utilised in their clinical roles.

The opportunity for a carefully considered personal review and application of some of these approaches seem to have been presented by the reflection strategy that is now an expectation of the revalidation process by the Nursing and Midwifery Council (NMC). The approach adopted for revalidation appears to exemplify the very structured procedures used to date by being based on evidencing five reflective pieces of work. While 'PREP' (Post-Registration Education & Practice) and the 'ENB (English National Board) portfolio' did not have a good record of success, the new NMC method provides an opportunity to embed reflective practice in nursing practice. Nurses are often now overheard saying, 'Note that for your portfolio,' and potential topics are also frequently explored in mentor updates as a basis for triennial review. Similarly, the NMC (2010) standards for pre-registration nursing education require nurses to be self-aware, evaluate their care and, importantly, learn by reflection as part of their personal and professional development. The Code 'will be central in the revalidation process as a focus for professional reflection'. (NMC, 2016: 6).

Using mnemonics and abridged models of reflection

Given the relative success of the use of mnemonics in clinical practice, such as the VERA communication framework in dementia care (Hawkes et al., 2015) and the adoption of the 'PICO' concept in research question formulation, the embracing of reflective techniques could be similarly aided by simplicity combined with approaches to reflection that are easy to learn and apply. Indeed, the limitations of staged models of reflection are acknowledged by Barksby et al. (2015), who instead advocate the use of the mnemonic 'Reflect' as a new model of reflection on action for clinical practice. Use of the mnemonic makes it easier than more traditional models of reflection (Table 6.2).

Similarly, Oelofsen (2012) proposes a 'reflective cycle' that has three simple stages:

- Step 1: *Curiosity* – This step involves noticing things, asking questions and questioning assumptions.
- Step 2: *Looking closer* – This step involves actively engaging with the questions from step 1.
- Step 3: *Transformation* – This phase is all about turning sense-making into action.

This framework was developed by the author when working with clinicians in different care contexts and from an interprofessional perspective. This approach can be used in facilitated groups or by individual practitioners in order to promote valuable reflective opportunities.

Another reflective technique – based on an abridged form of a model that could be utilised as a template – that provides simplicity and might be comparatively easy to use is the 'What?', 'So what?' and 'Now what?' process developed by Driscoll in 1994 (Table 6.3).

Table 6.2   'Reflect' as a new model of reflection on action for clinical practice

---

STAGE
(The REFLECT model comprises seven stages)

R – RECALL the events (Stage 1)
Give a brief overview of the situation upon which you are reflecting. This should consist of the facts – a description of what happened

E – EXAMINE your responses (Stage 2)
Discuss your thoughts and actions at the time of the incident upon which you are reflecting

F – Acknowledge FEELINGS (Stage 3)
Highlight any feelings you experienced at the time of the situation upon which you are reflecting

L – LEARN from the experience (Stage 4)
Highlight what you have learned from the situation

E – EXPLORE options (Stage 5)
Discuss options for the future if you were to encounter a similar situation

C – CREATE a plan of action (Stage 6)
Create a plan for the future - this can be for future theoretical learning or action

T – Set TIMESCALE (Stage 7)
Set a time by which the plan outlined in Stage 6 will be complete

---

By remembering the key questions in this way, this strategy promotes critical thinking in action on care situations aligned with the potential to make brief notes as soon as the opportunity becomes available. This approach can be useful as a structure for serious incident debriefing, biographical work, learning seminars or for clinical supervision.

Table 6.3   'What?', 'So what?' and 'Now what?' process, developed by Driscoll (1994)

Reflective Log
What? (A description of the event)
So what? (An analysis of the event)
Now what? (Proposed actions following the event)

Re-conceptualising reflective practice by applying 'black box' thinking to clinical nursing and service improvement

The importance of 'black box' thinking, based on the systematic method of investigating airline disasters, has recently been documented in a book by Syed (2016). The 'black box' refers to the plane's data recorder that is used after a crash in order to help investigate the cause. Syed (ibid.) states that aviation has an excellent safety record because, rather than being concealed, mistakes become learning opportunities. He explains that the concept is not concerned with literally creating a black box but, rather, with the 'willingness and tenacity to investigate the lessons that often exist when we fail, but which we rarely exploit' (ibid.: 165). He further describes how it is also about 'creating systems and cultures that enable organisations to learn from errors, rather than being threatened by them' (ibid.: 116). To emphasise his concept and the importance of resilience, determination and conceptual thinking, Syed describes how Sir James Dyson developed 5127 prototypes before his vacuum cleaner was finally ready to go on sale! He also explains how an anaesthetist worked with a nurse to overrule a surgeon who was incorrectly convinced that a patient was not experiencing an allergic reaction to latex and how junior Korean pilots were reluctant for cultural reasons to challenge more senior pilots, hence creating opportunities for error. As Syed explains, 'when we are confronted with evidence that challenges our deeply held beliefs we are more likely to reframe the evidence than we are to alter our beliefs' (ibid.: 375) (Table 6.4).

Table 6.4　The four key concepts that underpin 'black box' thinking

The use of factors that give marginal gain	Marginal gain is not concerned with implementing minor changes but in deconstructing a major problem into smaller components to determine what is effective and what does not work
Learning from mistakes	Developing procedures and cultures that facilitate organisational learning as opposed to concealment
Learning from successful organisations and individuals	The ability to be open to ideas and critical feedback and to be willing to learn from or share the outcomes of successful projects
Avoiding closed loops	Closed loops mean that mistakes are overlooked or misconstrued, whereas an open-loop system ensures action and progress

The notion of marginal gain

The 'notion of marginal gain' was employed to good effect in the Rio Olympics in 2016 in order to achieve the highest number of medals ever recorded by Team GB. The subtle or marginal gain techniques used included the use of the best available equipment and ergonomically designed apparel. Could such relatively minor changes have had a significant impact on athlete performance? It would appear so. It seems to the author that 'black box' thinking may well have potential relevance to healthcare and, hence, could be used for service improvement by following a similar methodical, yet reflective, structure. This method is not entirely dissimilar to established approaches to service improvement, whereby staff (often students) are encouraged to look for and highlight subtle changes in the care environment that could potentially have a significant impact on quality of care. Such changes or approaches to reflection have, for example, resulted in the more productive use of hand gel, which has reduced staff sickness rates, the provision of a clock in an operating theatre in order to ensure that hand-scrubbing conforms to procedures and Wi-Fi availability to promote the more efficient use of care plans in handovers.

The inability to learn from mistakes

The inability to learn from mistakes is based on cognitive dissonance, whereby, if errors occur, then these become difficult to admit to and so are often disregarded or subconsciously re-evaluated. Indeed, de Vries and Timmins (2015) have explained how poor practice, which they called 'care erosion', can result from a lack of effective reflective practice. To help overcome this phenomenon, they applied cognitive dissonance theory to several care situations. This theory explains how, when individuals become aware of inconsistencies, they experience discomfort (dissonance) between their thinking and behaviour. People are then motivated to react to remove the dissonance. De Vries and Timmins go on to explain how three focal points to address care erosion emerge from the application of dissonance theory:

- *Improve (or restore) the effectiveness of critical reflection* – By 'reflecting in a methodical way, aimed at practice improvement'.
- *Promote and maintain strong values and standards* – 'The nurse needs to become aware of the practical impact of strong values and their expression in practice and their potential to cause dissonance.'
- *Promote optimal care and awareness of signs of care erosion* – 'Care erosion can be avoided if early signs are addressed before contagion and conformity create its slippery slope.' (Ibid.: 7)

The 'ability to learn from successful individuals' is exemplified in the following case study, combined with the potential of the application of black box thinking to nursing.

Avoiding closed loops

Much of the published literature on communication in nursing is about using closed-loop systems so as to prevent unnecessary risks or misunderstanding. Therefore, a warning that consideration of the use of open-loop systems might cause

Case Study 6.1   Jamie's Story

Jamie was working as a newly qualified nurse in a community dementia team. The team already offered people recently diagnosed with dementia the opportunity to compile their life story. Because of the author's request to think about his reflective practice, 'J' noted that the uptake of life-story work by people with dementia had declined over the past year. 'J' spoke to clinicians experienced in life-story work and read publications by nurses who had compiled their life story and then shared this with relatives and service users before inviting them to develop their biographies. The impact of this was to demonstrate a commitment to the concept of life-story work and to show how powerful it could be. It also promoted a positive therapeutic relationship with the person and their family and an increase in the number of individuals undertaking life-story work. While not apparently a reflective approach, the careful use of evidence and consultation to re-evaluate a care strategy enabled an improvement in life-story uptake and potentially enhanced the quality of care.

cognitive dissonance! Syed (2016) explains that an open-loop system is concerned with implementing a strategy, then testing if it has been successful, working on any presenting problems, thereby enhancing the strategy.

Perhaps consider this idea in respect of your own health/social care organisation or NHS Trust and reflect on the structures that exist to support nurses to speak out about patient safeguarding concerns. Such a requirement is part of your professional code of conduct. Does your organisation facilitate such a culture? Are staff supported to raise concerns? Perhaps make notes on any examples of good practice that you come up with or, equally, any areas that require improvement.

Clearly, the notion of 'black box' thinking has resonated with the author of this chapter. I am of the view that the fundamental concepts outlined above have applicability to nursing and should be utilised and tested in the clinical setting. That said, often, the sheer pace of and pressures in practice, mitigate against taking time for even the briefest critical reviews of care situations. However, this chapter has established that the use of the 'black box' thinking phenomenon could help resolve some quality of care problems. One potential approach that could also be tested in such situations is an idea closely allied to the notion of marginal gain, namely 'one-minute' interaction analysis.

Activity 6.3   Reflective Exercise

Perhaps test this idea out. Take just a minute or two to step back from the intensity of your clinical role and observe an interaction between a colleague and a patient in your practice environment. What communication techniques is your colleague employing? Is the person being listened to in a meaningful way? What non-verbal signals are being given?

Creating opportunities for 'bringing the mind home'

It seems to the author that removing oneself from stressful situations and taking the time to contemplate is essential. Is it similar to Johns' notion of bringing the mind home by making space for reflection? While compiling this chapter, I spoke to a number of qualified nurses about how they create opportunities for reflection and have recorded below the ideas that they found to be both useful and efficient. Essentially, these strategies are concerned with opportunities for reflection in action, however, as has been seen, establishing a time for reflection on action can be equally important.

··

Activity 6.4   Reflective Exercise

Ask some of your practice colleagues if they reflect and, if they do so, how they go about it.

Emphasise that this exercise isn't concerned with trying to catch them out but with documenting the creative ways in which reflection can take place. The approaches used by your colleagues may include making notes and thinking about everyday practice activities in a different way.

Make a bullet point list of the reflective techniques that they use. Are any of them useful for your own practice?

··

A popular method seems to be keeping a notebook to hand and then later using these records to make an entry into a personal journal. Both can take advantage of the abridged headings from established or new models of reflection. Some nurses have extended this idea by using a Dictaphone or audio device to record personal thoughts for a later discussion or portfolio entry, but, again, you may need to check local information governance procedures if you plan to use this approach. The logical progression from a journal is to consider the use of tablet computers, apps or other software, interactive whiteboards, work-supplied mobile phones or laptops. Again, information-governance procedures will need to be checked. These means are already being used to record care events, so why not use your mobile device to note your reflections? Meanwhile, Knight (2015) explains how a facilitated reflective practice group, based on containment principles, enables participants to express their thoughts in a form that is more meaningful and endurable. The structure of these groups is provided by agreeing on ground rules, promoting positive conversation and by broadly using the framework of a reflective model.

Some adult nursing colleagues cited the use of 'bedside handovers' as events for reflective practice and learning opportunities. Additionally, many mental health nurses spoke of the usefulness of clinical supervision as occasions for reflection. Most talked about the importance of individual supervision but a number mentioned group supervision because this was more realistic regarding resources. The use of recording in the 'first person' in care plans was cited as a means of promoting care ownership by service users. In turn, this enables empowerment and contributes to recovery. Structured storytelling has been used to promote engagement. Brief seminars on clinical issues based on Driscoll's work was also mentioned and so, too, was case formulation, which is a process that promotes reflective practice and critical discussion in mental health, which then increases clinician understanding of and empathy towards service users. The starting point for this is often the consideration of the person's life story. Case Study 6.2 gives an example of how case formulation might be used to support reflective practice and so contribute to the professional revalidation requirements.

Case Study 6.2   Parveen's Story

Parveen, an experienced charge nurse working in an acute mental health inpatient unit, found the pressure of working in such an environment demanding, particularly regarding finding the time to document care events and risk management. Parveen was aware of the value of reflection in terms of enhancing her use of evidence-based practice and the need for professional development. She suggested that a way of still meeting her personal aims of using an integrative approach to reflection was to utilise a case-formulation style within scheduled ward handover meetings. This consisted of using a personal biographical approach as a precursor to discussing service user needs. The outcome of this process was detailed written entries in care records, which then promoted a more meaningful and individualised dialogue with service users. This also provided the basis for entry into Parveen's NMC revalidation portfolio.

Conclusion

This chapter has acknowledged the pressures inherent in contemporary clinical practice but has emphasised the positive personal and care outcomes of making time for reflection. The focus has been on describing a number of creative approaches to reflection that aimed to provide a chapter that you could 'dip in and out of'. Many of these ideas have been suggested by clinicians, while some have been published in academic papers. The strategies for reflection include the use of mnemonics or abridged models of reflection-on-action, re-conceptualising reflection by utilising the principles of 'black box' thinking, marginal gain and cognitive dissonance theory and by outlining several approaches that create opportunities for 'bringing the mind home'.

The author hopes that you will test out some of these ideas and incorporate them into your practice. It may be that you develop your own eclectic paradigm of reflection by taking the best parts of each approach or strategy to fit with the uniqueness of your experiences. Good luck with the methods that you use. Please bear in mind that reflection does not have to be on negative or difficult situations, reflect on the positive things, too.

References

Barksby, J., Butcher, N. and Whysall, A. (2015) 'A new model of reflection for clinical practice', *Nursing Times, 111*, (34/35): 21–3.

Boud, D., Keogh, R. and Walker, D. (1985) *Reflection: Turning Experience into Learning.* London: Kogan Page.

Bulman, C., and Schutz, S. (2013) *Reflective Practice in Nursing.* Chichester: Blackwell.

Caldwell, L. and Grobbel, C. (2013) 'The importance of reflective practice in nursing', *International Journal of Caring Sciences, 6* (3): 319–26.

Carper, B.A. (1978) 'Fundamental patterns of knowing in nursing', *Advances in Nursing Science, 1* (1): 13–24.

de Vries, J. and Timmins, F. (2015) 'Care erosion in hospitals: Problems in reflective nursing practice and the role of cognitive dissonance', *Nurse Education Today, 38*: 5–8.

Driscoll, J. (1994) 'Reflective practice for practise', *Senior Nurse, 13* (Jan/Feb): 47–50.

Gibbs, G. (1988) *Learning by Doing: A Guide to Teaching and Learning Methods.* Oxford: Further Education Unit, Oxford Brookes University.

Hawkes, D., Hingley, D., Wood, S. and Blackhall, A. (2015) 'Evaluating the VERA Framework', *Nursing Standard Art and Science, 30* (2): 44–8.

Jasper, M. (2013) *Beginning Reflective Practice.* Hampshire: Cengage Learning.

Johns, C. (1995) 'Framing learning through reflection within Carper's fundamental ways of knowing in nursing', *Journal of Advanced Nursing, 22* (2): 226–34.

Knight, S. (2015) 'Realising the benefits of reflective practice', *Nursing Times, 111* (23/24): 7–19.

Kolb, D.A. (1984) *Experiential Learning: Experience as the Source of Learning and Development.* Upper Saddle River, NJ: Prentice-Hall.

Nursing and Midwifery Council (NMC) (2010) *Standards for Pre-registration Nursing Education.* London: NMC.

NMC (2016) *The Code: Professional Standards of Practice and Behaviour for Nurses and Midwives.* London: NMC.

Oelofsen, N. (2012) 'Using reflective practice in frontline nursing', *Nursing Times, 108* (24): 22–4.

Schön, D.A. (1983) *The Reflective Practitioner.* London: Temple Smith.

Schön, D.A. (1987) *Educating the Reflective Practitioner: Toward a New Design for Teaching and Learning in the Professions.* San Francisco, CA: Jossey-Bass.

Syed, M. (2016) *Black Box Thinking: Marginal Gains and the Secrets of High Performance.* London: John Murray.

Tashiro, J., Shimpuku, Y., Naruse, K. and Matsutani, M. (2013) 'Concept analysis of reflection in nursing professional development', *Japan Journal of Nursing Science, 10*: 170–9.

7

Self-Compassion

Tess Wagstaffe and Ness Woodcock-Dennis

But how shall we expect charity towards others, when we are uncharitable to ourselves? 'Charity begins at home,' is the voice of the world; yet is every man his greatest enemy, and as it were, his own executioner. (Sir Thomas Browne, 1642, in Wilkin, 1846: 96)

Chapter aims

- Introduce self-compassion.
- Discuss the benefits of self-compassion.
- Explore some of the barriers to self-compassion.
- Explore how we can be self-compassionate in challenging clinical situations, 'when things go wrong'.
- Suggest some activities to promote the cultivation of self-compassion.

Introduction

Our job as nurses is to care for others experiencing vulnerability and distress. We are trained to deliver compassionate person-centred care in environments that are not always conducive to this expectation. Aside from being highly skilled, clinically competent practitioners, nurses are often expected to have answers and solve problems, not only for those in our care, but for our colleagues, too. Whilst the focus of healthcare should be patient-orientated, the demands on nurses in the current healthcare climate are increasing. In this chapter, we will introduce the concept of 'self-compassion' and look at how nurses can explore and develop self-care practices.

It is perhaps not surprising that a recent focus on the importance of compassion and self-compassion within nursing and other healthcare professions is focused on patient outcomes. Self-compassion is often explored in terms of how it can improve patient care (Gustin and Wagner, 2013) rather than focusing on the benefits for the individual nurse or on nursing as a community. Whilst it is important that nurses focus and reflect on improving the quality of care that they deliver, it is also important that when considering self-compassion, the focus is at least equally in exploring its impact on improving the quality of the nurse's experience within their role and within their life.

It has been argued that nurses need to be able to experience self-compassion in order to be compassionate towards those they care for. There are many nurses who would probably describe feeling that they can deliver compassionate care despite struggling with self-compassion. Whilst the mutuality of this dynamic can be a subject for discussion, the main concern of this chapter is to explore how we, as nurses, can be compassionate to ourselves.

What is self-compassion?

Being self-compassionate means that you aim to be happy and healthy in the long term. It means treating yourself with warmth and understanding in times of stress, failure and suffering. Instead of 'beating ourselves up' over the things that we failed to do, being self-compassionate allows us to recognise our imperfections and the inevitability of difficult life experiences. Being self-compassionate is about being easier on yourself when you experience hardship, rather than feeling angry and self-critical. The problem is that the culture of healthcare sets a firm expectation, which, when organisations are under-resourced, becomes unrealistic, however this is built into the nursing psyche, and when as nurses we reject this reality, we experience frustration and our own suffering. If we can learn to accept this reality with empathy and kindness, then we are more likely to feel calmer and emotionally composed in the face of adversity.

Neff (2003: 89) states that the concept of self-compassion is an extension of compassion but compassion that is extended to ourselves, and defines three important components of self-compassion as (Figure 7.1):

Self-kindness

extending kindness and understanding to oneself rather than harsh judgement and self-criticism

Common humanity

Seeing one's experiences as part of the larger human experience rather than seeing them as separating and isolating

Mindfulness

Holding one's painful thoughts and feelings in balanced awareness rather than over identifying with them

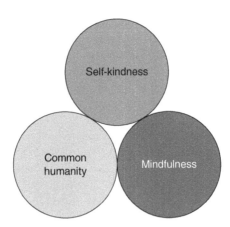

Figure 7.1   The components of compassion (Neff, 2003: 89), reproduced with permission of Taylor & Francis

Whilst these concepts may make sense intellectually, the reality of applying such principles to ourselves whilst we are caught up in the anxiety and emotional overload of caring work can appear to be unrealistic. This can leave us with a sense of frustration and failure when our expectations are not met. However, the benefits of caring for ourselves on a deeper emotional level are numerous (Germer, 2009; Neff, 2015).

In a study exploring nurses' personal dignity and self-esteem, Sturm and Dellert (2016) noted that, whilst nurses commonly identify the importance of dignity, it is as a 'component of the patients' experience rather than as necessarily in the nurses own lives' (ibid.: 1). We believe that this is currently the same with compassion, that as nurses we are more familiar with understanding compassion either in relation to how we can extend this to our service users or in term of how we can use self-compassion to improve their experience. We can acknowledge the importance of compassion but are unable to see the necessity of it in our own lives.

Being non-judgemental, respecting human vulnerability and creating a healing environment are all important components of compassionate care. Yet, are we able to respect our own vulnerability, approach our own fallibility with kindness and patience, speak up for ourselves when it is necessary, or are these compassionate tasks, tasks that we can only carry out for others who are in receipt of our care?

If we consider ourselves in a holistic way, often we are quick to notice physical injury as it is often more easily identified through its manifestation of pain and, usually as individuals, we attend to this quickly. Are we as likely to offer the same attention to psychological and emotional pain? It is suggested that the role of emotion is overlooked in healthcare settings, particularly the emotions of healthcare workers (Robichaud, 2003).

If we consider prophylactic routines to ensure maintenance of physical health such as brushing our teeth to maintain oral health or health-screening interventions, it is possible to protect our emotional health further through this concept through daily practices known to contribute to resilience. We will be exploring which routines can be incorporated in order to promote self-care and self-compassion, aimed at empowering you to support your own well-being.

The benefits of self-compassion

Consider a time when a friend was in distress. It is almost certain that most of us respond to a friend's distress with kindness and genuine concern, but how often do we respond with kindness to our own distress? Responding with compassion to our own pain and distress brings many benefits. It is suggested that self-compassion improves well-being as it assists individuals in feeling connected, cared for and emotionally calmer (Gilbert, 2005).

Being compassionate to ourselves is often overlooked, particularly when our identity is as a nurse. This is largely due to the nature of the nursing profession and caring organisations: in other words, putting others first has become a cultural component of nurse's identity. However, most of us have many roles outside of nursing. If we consider ourselves beyond the nursing identity, the conditions for self-compassion may be more conducive.

Much is written on the need for nurses to develop emotional resilience, particularly in response to reducing burnout and the negative effects associated with the emotional labour of caring. Studies have shown that nurses who have higher levels of self-compassion experience lower levels of burnout and, as a result, have an increased capacity to demonstrate compassion to others (Durkin et al., 2016; Duarte et al., 2016). The correlation between self-compassion and capacity for compassion to others is not unique to UK nurses. International studies are beginning to indicate that this is a significant issue within nursing (Heffernan et al., 2010) and a way of fostering genuine compassion (Mills et al., 2015). This is possibly contentious for some nurses. For many, their experience will be that they do not feel a lack of compassion for those whom they care for. Feelings of failure accompanying a feeling that have been unable to alleviate the suffering of others can lead to harsh and critical judgement of themselves.

If we consider physical well-being, studies reveal that individuals who are self-compassionate experience better mental health – specifically, they are more likely to be resilient, happier and optimistic (Neff, 2017).

Part of the reason for this is down to the processes of our emotional brain. When we can soothe ourselves, we release the hormone oxytocin. Known as the love hormone, this chemical plays a vital role in the formation of social bonds. The more oxytocin we release, the more likely it is that we are kinder to ourselves; it has a synergistic effect on our well-being and is a virtuous process (Gerhardt, 2015).

Oxytocin production is stimulated by physical touch. It is an innate human response to soothe those in distress whom we care about. When babies cry, as parents we soothe and hold them close to our hearts. New parents are encouraged to hold their babies *skin to skin* to encourage bonding; this stimulates the production of oxytocin and protects the immune system (ibid.). When adults whom we care for are distressed, in Western cultures our response is often to hug them and provide comfort and reassurance through touch. Touch reduces cortisol (the stress hormone) and increases oxytocin.

The combination of oxytocin and social support has shown increased resilience in individuals through reduced levels of cortisol and anxiety (Heinrichs et al., 2003).

Neff's research suggests that self-compassion is also a prompt for the production of oxytocin.

The Problems of Avoidance

> We measure our happiness by the gap between what we want and how things are. (Germer, 2009: 12)

One of the biggest barriers to self-compassion is our own expectation. The work of Christopher Germer suggests that our failure to successfully execute approaches are down to our own motivation and confusion about how our minds work. For example, when we feel good, we fail to recognise the need to maintain feeling good; in other words, we behave reactively, dealing with problems when they become a problem, as opposed to taking a proactive stance in which we would consider maintaining good feeling.

It is suggested that the definition of 'acceptance' is to: 'embrace whatever arises within us, moment to moment, just as it is' (ibid.: 11). However, we instinctively reject uncomfortable feelings that create dissonance between reality and our expectations, creating a feeling of dissatisfaction, a notion central to Buddhism referred to as 'Dhukha', often described as 'suffering' or 'un-satisfactoriness' (Sangharakshita, 1990: 93) and, yet, in fact, is more aligned with the definition of 'deep, subtle sense of dissatisfaction that is a part of every mind moment and that results directly from the mental treadmill' (Gunaratana, 2002: 11). Similarly, Gilbert and Choden (2013) refer to this as the 'disappointment gap' between our 'actual self' and our 'undesired self' and our vulnerability as individuals to shame and self-criticism. This is an extended aspect of the role-expectation plays, as quite often we experience discomfort as a result of how we perceive what others think of us. Negative perceptions are harmful. Rumination becomes self-criticism and self-attacking. This process does nothing to serve us, as this behaviour is threat focussed, which keeps our stress response active.

Often, in turning away from pain, we adopt dysfunctional mechanisms to reduce stress, such as manifestation of unhealthy behaviours such as comfort-eating (Germer, 2009) or use of intoxicants. A study by Gibbons et al. (2010) focuses on the relationship between causes of stress and emotional well-being in student nurses. The findings suggest that avoidance-coping is a predictor in a decline of emotional well-being, and that dispositional control and positive strategies to support self-efficacy are likely to impact well-being positively.

The Working Environment as a Barrier

The current reality of nursing in the UK continues to present challenges. Provisional statistics reveal that 'work–life balance' is the main reason cited for staff leaving the

NHS (NHS Digital, 2017). Increased organisational demands are placing individuals under enormous pressure, leading to workplace stress and dissatisfaction in the workplace and can affect nurses' ability to deliver compassionate care as they feel overstretched both physically and emotionally. Considering these factors, it is likely that self-compassion becomes even less of a consideration for nurses.

Barratt (2017) suggests that it is the responsibility of employing organisations to improve support for staff as a means of fostering a climate of compassionate care for staff and patients. It is not the sole responsibility of healthcare professionals to individually find ways to cope with the challenging context in which they work.

On a positive note, organisations are beginning to recognise the need for more compassionate practices for staff, and in many settings are beginning to respond with proactive measures, such as the introduction of Schwartz Rounds (Point of Care Foundation, 2017) and of Mindfulness-Based Cognitive Therapy (MBCT) (Graham, 2014), seeing significant improvements in participating NHS staff, in terms of well-being and reduced sickness. Whilst these interventions are not directly about self-compassion and do not address resource and political issues such as current staffing issues, they do offer staff opportunities through developing these practices to improve their well-being, and signal the importance of self-care.

Self-Compassion vs Guilt and Self-Criticism

Whilst many of us struggle with self-compassion in everyday situations, perhaps a greater challenge is how we develop self-compassion even when we feel that we have failed in a clinical situation. Clinical mistakes, or perceived misjudgements, can be devastating and life-changing for clinicians, service users and families. Whilst our experiences of coping will be different, depending on individual personalities, is it possible to cultivate a compassionate attitude towards ourselves under these difficult circumstances? Many of us may be able to relate to feelings of guilt when we feel that we have not provided the care that ideally we would like to provide for a variety of reasons within clinical situations.

Barron et al. (2017) explored mental health nurses' interpretations and expectations of compassion. They describe nurses feeling as though 'The weight is on their shoulders' (ibid.: 217) and nurses experiencing guilt when tasks were forgotten or they felt as though they were not practising compassionately. One participant in the study spoke of not knowing how to survive through the anxiety-provoking and intense nature of nursing. Not getting things right can present in many forms, from serious clinical incidents to our self-criticism over everyday interactions that we feel were not good enough. Not being able to deliver the care we aim for due to time/resource pressures can also cause us to feel that we have let our service users down.

This may lead us to question how we can cope with the shame and guilt that we sometimes experience and the punitive self-criticism that we then may experience. Whilst it is a recognisable requirement of compassion to be non-judgemental, how can we extend this to ourselves? It can feel really difficult or even impossible.

Many of the texts on self-compassion discuss our propensity to be self-critical (Gilbert and Choden, 2013) and the frustration, depression and withdrawal that this can cause, it can be hard as a clinician to relate to the texts that refer to errors that are probably not life-changing for others, like those that we may experience in the clinical settings. Fears and anxieties around not getting everything right in clinical practice can leave us feeling anxious, isolated and scared.

How can we move away from the feelings of guilt and self-criticism? In what way does the guilt and self-criticism serve us? Experiencing feelings of guilt and failure is a unifying phenomenon for all of us. Probably most of us do not share these feelings with our peers and hence we can feel a sense of isolation.

If we consider the context suggested by Gilbert and Choden (2013), then it is vital to identify sources of self-criticism because ruminating on our shortcomings and less desirable aspects of ourselves is not only unhelpful, but also damaging as it keeps us trapped in the past, which cannot be changed. Self-compassion does not suggest not improving. In fact, it is the 'shame-based self-attacking' (Gilbert, 2013: 373) that rarely opens up an opportunity for personal growth. In fact, at times, it can paralyse us. The potentially consuming angst can lead to avoidance behaviour and severely diminishes our satisfaction in the workplace. So, how can some of these barriers be addressed? We shall draw on Neff's (2003) three components by applying real practice examples (Scenario 7.1).

Scenario 7.1

You have returned home after a late shift. You are running half an hour late and, on the drive home, you play details of the shift over in your head. You feel frustrated as you recall how busy the shift was. You feel angry that you are expected to run a shift that is understaffed. You feel that there was not enough time to sit with a service user who was particularly distressed and worry as to whether everyone's care plans and risk assessments are up to date. It feels impossible to switch off and you feel stressed and anxious ...

Most of us can relate to the above scenario. An important question to ask yourself is how you relax following a stressful shift. Many of us adopt coping mechanisms in order to deal with our mind replaying the frustrating details but, what is often not considered is the lack of attention that we give to our physiology in such moments. If we are to consider the stress hormones that we experience so as to enable us to perform in challenging situations, we may be more likely to consider ourselves with kindness.

On returning from such a stressful shift, it is likely that we may have not had an opportunity to eat a meal or even to have a drink, yet, as nurses, we are aware of the importance of adequate hydration and nourishment to regulate our body systems such as the impact of dehydration and low blood sugar levels on our mental functioning. Shifts such as these are likely to be made even more stressful by interactions with other people who are stressed. When these factors are combined with our own 'flight-or-fight' stress response, it is not difficult to understand why we might end the day anxious or angry. When we can consider our experience in physiological terms, we are more likely to understand the proactive measures that we can take to assist to protect ourselves.

To enable self-compassion, it is important to understand that it is different to self-indulgence and self-pity. Neff (2017) describes self-indulgent behaviours as unbalanced and potentially harmful in the long term. We agree that well-being is at risk from overindulgence. This might manifest as drinking too much alcohol or overeating. We may overindulge through constant rumination following stressful shifts or days at work. We may find that we feel sorry for ourselves, adopting a mindset of 'Why me?', 'Why do I always get the stressful shift?' Such patterns rarely alleviate our feeling of suffering in the long term, and can become addictive and harmful very quickly, by which self-pitying behaviours occur.

Self-pitying behaviours contract the world around us, isolating us from others, and lead to feelings of resentment. It is a negative cycle and a place of stagnation, where things become 'stuck'. Self-pity comprises of self-hatred and poor self-esteem. It disables us from taking responsibility and is perpetuated by the belief that there is 'nothing we can do about it' (Germer, 2009; Mason-John and Groves, 2013).

Taking physiology into consideration, we know that drinking alcohol excessively is counterproductive as it acts as a depressant. Similarly, products containing caffeine will serve only to heighten anxiety as they act as a stimulant. This is a small example. However, when we are able to think about the details, we open up the way to become empowered to plan choices that will serve us, as opposed to quick fixes that keep us trapped in a potentially harmful cycle.

Activity 7.1   Reflective Practice

Reflect on how you may react and behave following a stressful or difficult day at work. Are there any changes that you could make that would better reflect an attitude of kindness towards yourself? This could entail changing behaviours or incorporating new behaviours into your routine. Try and visualise how this would look and how you may feel if you make these changes.

   If you choose to, next time you return from work following a difficult day, put the above idea into practice and see if you feel that you have demonstrated a sense of compassion towards yourself.

The concept of community is also a central feature of the work of Ballatt and Campling (2015), who suggest the importance of the role of kinship among healthcare staff if they are to enhance compassion toward one another and patients in their care. This element of self-compassion entails knowing that suffering, and at times feeling inadequate, is a shared human experience, as opposed to one that is experienced by us alone. At a recent nursing conference in Finland, a colleague from the Netherlands stated:

De kinderen van de kapper zijn slecht geknipt. (Translated as: 'The barber's child's hair is badly cut.'

It became apparent that many international nursing colleagues had similar anecdotes, confirming that healthcare professionals from a variety of disciplines and cultures also have difficulty in caring for themselves.

Self-care is a skill that is learned through social interaction and role-modelling. However, if we view our own suffering in isolation, as opposed to recognising it as a mutual phenomenon, we are more likely to fall into self-pity. Neff (2017) defines common humanity as a vital aspect of self-compassion, as compassion means to 'suffer with', implying that it is a universal human experience to experience pain and failure.

It is a common experience to focus on ourselves in times of stress and vulnerability, even blaming ourselves, however if we learn to connect to our common humanity, then we are less likely to be myopic in terms of our feelings and, in turn, to be less self-critical as we can recognise that everyone at some point will experience feelings of failure and inadequacy.

Nevertheless, clinical workplace environments can be hostile and ultimately work against the cultivation of kinship. It is the individual responsibility of everyone to cultivate a compassionate culture through role-modelling compassionate behaviours on a humanitarian level through mindful interaction with individuals, irrespective of professional status and experience. A Finnish study of student nurses' views of loving-caring in nurse education found students describing 'caring' as an internal experience of authenticity and 'motivation to help' and being able to consider humans to be similar to oneself, irrespective of gender, age, race or status (Paldanius and Maatta, 2011). However, this is challenging within societal constraints (Mamgain, 2010), particularly in institutions that lack compassion and are 'driven by crisis – where there is little time for reflection' (Waddington, 2016: 5). Yet, these attributes are desperately required for developing resilience and managing stress (Bright et al., 2016).

In the context of nursing culture, Ballatt supports this view by stating that: 'The contents of the environment, influences the growth of the contents' (2016), further describing the lack of acknowledgement around healthcare staff experiences of culturally entrenched ineffective group dynamics as 'scandalous' (ibid.).

Role-modelling is a key component of nursing (NMC, 2017; RCN, 2017). The damaging power of negative role-modelling is recognised, along with the need for kindness to be valued (Ballatt and Campling, 2015). Genuinely valuing and appreciating our colleagues is vital to fostering a culture of compassion because: 'Caring also manifests itself in nurse's interaction' (Paldanius and Maatta, 2011: 86). A positive culture is essential for nurses to deliver person-centred compassionate care, as culture shapes the way in which healthcare practitioners work (Hewitt-Taylor, 2015).

A vital aspect of positive role-modelling to change culture by leaders authentically is by acknowledging vulnerability (Armstrong, 2016). By inspiring others to be self-compassionate about their flaws, greater self-awareness can be gained (Neff, 2003), which is required for emotionally intelligent strengths-based leadership (NMC, 2017; Vesterinen et al., 2012), as a correlation is suggested between emotional intelligence and self-compassion (Senyuva et al., 2014).

When considering self-compassion and the workplace, Barron et al. (2017) consider two important elements in how individuals managed their levels of compassion and self-compassion. This involved looking after one another and also being aware of life pressures outside of work and how these affect compassion. Whilst much of this study focused on the development of compassionate practice rather than self-compassion, the study highlights the importance of a supportive team, the informal supervision processes, listening to one another and through peer support identifying when work–life balance is an issue.

The study also acknowledged how levels of compassion can be affected by issues of transference that sometimes we will work with service users whose situations or life experiences will affect us emotionally. This can affect our ability to be compassionate to that person or to ourselves. Sometimes, we may experience feelings of self-hatred or poor self-esteem due to these negative feelings towards our service users. How do we seek support when this may be the case for us?

Viewing this through a perspective of common humanity, we can acknowledge that others have experiences of similar difficulties and conflicts. We may choose (if we feel that we are working within a supportive environment) to share these difficulties with others. This may help us gain different perspectives. It may mean that work is reallocated or that our peers offer us suggestions as to how to work differently in this situation. If may simply allow us a chance for catharsis and feeling listened to.

If you feel that our workplace does not offer this support, is there other peer support available, for example through mentoring or clinical supervision? Creating an environment that nurtures positive professional relationships not only strengthens resilience but is also, or can be, an expression of self-care that emanates from a self-compassionate stance. Mentoring or clinical supervision can provide an essential support network and a safe place in which to explore concerns, share fears, challenge ourselves and grow. Essential to this process is choosing a supervisor or mentor who is supportive and whose 'style' of mentoring suits you. Whilst it is undoubtedly difficult to fit in the time for supervision, it can provide an invaluable, nurturing, supportive space (Case Study 7.1).

Case Study 7.1

I was working in quite a complex and difficult clinical environment and, following major changes to the staff group I felt unsupported, stressed and anxious. I tried to discuss this with my manager but was unable to gain any support. Neither did I feel that I was connecting with any of my new colleagues to either offer or receive support. I went outside of the workplace and arranged clinical supervision with a past colleague, who I trusted and respected. This offered me the space to explore how to address the difficulties I was facing at work. Whilst it was not easy to arrange the time to do this, this support really helped me contain the anxiety I was experiencing and helped me to seek solutions to some of the problems I was facing.

Another option is to think about how we create spaces for connectedness and common humanity with our peers and colleagues. This could involve contemplating whether there is space in handover to discuss cases that we perceive as difficult and challenging, or thinking about whether Schwartz Rounds could be an option within the workplace.

Mindfulness

In developing self-compassion, we attempt to approach our emotions in a balanced way, to avoid suppressing or exaggerating any aspects of our experience. By teaching ourselves to *observe* our experiences, both internally and externally, as they are, we are able to see our situation from a broader perspective. By adopting a non-judgemental state of mind, which is cultivated by mindfulness practice, we learn to see our emotions as they are and be less likely to be caught up in over-analysis and negative reactivity.

In the previous chapter, mindfulness and how this can be applied to our nursing practice has been explored at length. Mindfulness can help us to improve our ability to pay attention to our thoughts and feelings and to try and observe them without the usual judgements or criticisms that we sometimes apply to our thought processes. Applying the mindfulness practices as suggested in chapter can therefore help us to lessen these judgements and criticisms and to become less attached to them. Having this more balanced perspective can also help us to perhaps take action where it is needed as we are less caught up and distracted with our emotional attachment to the situation (Activity 7.2).

· ·

Activity 7.2

Identify a time to consider ways in which you can develop self-compassion using the three different components. It would be a good idea to allocate a period of time to each component separately:

- Self-kindness

  Consider any changes that you could make that would reflect an attitude of kindness towards yourself. This could entail changing behaviours or incorporating new behaviours into your routine. Whilst these could be as simplistic as self-care such as a relaxing bath, it could also involve bigger changes such as incorporating clinical supervision into your worklife or consulting with occupational health if you feel that your health is being affected by work.

- Mindfulness

  Review Chapter 5 on 'Nursing and Mindfulness' and consider the exercises and whether you could incorporate one of these into your weekly or daily routine. You could consider downloading a mindfulness app or build the 'pause' into part of your daily routine.

- Common humanity

Are there any forums that you could participate in within the workplace or even consider developing (incorporating one into handover, for example) that could develop the sense of connectedness with work colleagues? Could you become involved in a Schwartz Round? Are there smaller everyday interactions with colleagues that could enhance your sense of connectedness?

Conclusion

Organisations can feel like unyielding and hostile environments in which to work. As nurses, it is often easier to identify with the importance of compassion in relation to the importance of demonstrating this towards our service users. These factors can present challenges to the cultivation and nurturing of compassionate behaviours towards ourselves.

It is important to develop self-compassion because the nature of nursing work can diminish it. We are worthy of it and should not feel exposed to relentless criticism and self-criticism, nor to feel a sense of isolation and failure. We are worthy of kindness, soothing and connectedness with others. We merit the healing that we wish for our patients and service users. Whilst not turning away from reflection, self-improvement (if that is what we feel that we need) or challenging ourselves, we should strive to approach this with kindness, gentleness and patience when this is what is required.

References

Armstrong, A. (2016) Compassion in Organisations, Compassion, Organisational Change and the Future of Care, Compassion Conference, University of Essex, 2/9/17.

Ballatt, J. (2016) Compassion, Organisational Change and the Future of Care, Compassion Conference, University of Essex, 2/9/17.

Ballatt, J. and Campling, P. (2015) *Intelligent Kindness: Reforming the Culture of Healthcare.* London: Royal College of Psychiatrists.

Barratt, C. (2017) 'Exploring how mindfulness and self-compassion can enhance compassionate care', *Nursing Standard*, 31: 55–62.

Barron, K., Deery, R. and Sloan, G. (2017) '"Community mental health nurses" and compassion: An interpretative approach', *Journal of Psychiatric & Mental Health Nursing*, 24: 211–20.

Bright, J., Eliahoo, R. and Pokorny, H. (2016) *Enhancing Teaching Practice in Higher Education* (ed. H. Pokorny and D. Warren). London: Sage.

Duarte, J., Pinto-Gouveia, J. and Cruz, B. (2016) 'Relationships between nurses' empathy, self-compassion and dimensions of professional quality of life: A cross-sectional study', *International Journal of Nursing Studies*, 60: 1–11.

Durkin, M., Beaumont, E., Hollins Martin C.J. and Carson, J. (2016) 'A pilot study exploring the relationship between self-compassion, self-judgement, self-kindness, compassion, professional quality of life and wellbeing among UK community nurses', *Nurse Education Today*, 46: 109–14.

Gerhardt, S. (2015) *Why Love Matters: How Affection Shapes a Baby's Brain.* Hove: Routledge.

Germer, C. (2009) *The Mindful Path to Self-Compassion: Freeing Yourself from Destructive Thoughts and Emotions.* New York: Guilford Press.

Gibbons, C., Dempster, M. and Moutray, M. (2010) 'Stress, coping and satisfaction in nursing students', *Journal of Advanced Nursing*, 67 (3): 621–32.

Gilbert, P. (2005) 'Compassion and cruelty: A biopsychosocial approach', in P. Gilbert (ed.), *Compassion: Conceptualisations, Research and Use in Psychotherapy.* London: Routledge.

Gilbert, P. (2013) *The Compassionate Mind.* London: Robinson.

Gilbert, P. and Choden (2013) Mindful Compassion, London: Robinson

Graham, L. (2014) *NHS Staff Mindfulness (MBCT) Project 2011 to 2014 Large Reductions in Staff Sickness Rates One Year Following MBCT Course.* Available at: www.nwppn.nhs.uk/attachments/article/660/Staff_Mindfulness_Project.pdf (accessed July 2017).

Gunaratana, B.H. (2002) *Mindfulness in Plain English.* Boston, MA: Wisdom, p. 11.

Gustin, L. and Wagner, L. (2013) 'The butterfly effect of caring: Clinical nursing teachers' understanding of self-compassion as a source to compassionate care', *Scandinavian Journal of Caring Sciences*, 27 (1): 175–83.

Heffernan, M., Quinn Griffin, M.T., McNulty, R. and Fitzpatrick, J.J. (2010) 'Self-compassion and emotional intelligence in nurses', *International Journal of Nursing Practice*, 16: 366–73.

Heinrichs, M., Baumgartner, T., Kirschbaum, C. and Ehlert, U. (2003) 'Social support and oxytocin interact to supress cortisol and subjective responses to psychological stress', *Biological Psychiatry*, 54: 1389–98.

Hewitt-Taylor, J. (2015) *Developing Person-Centred Practice: A Practical Approach to Quality Healthcare.* London: Palgrave.

Mamgain, V. (2010) 'Ethical consciousness in the classroom: how Buddhist practices can help develop empathy and compassion', *Journal of Transformative Education 8* (1): 22–41.

Mason-John, V. and Groves, P. (2013) *Eight Step Recovery.* Cambridge: Windhorse.

McDonald, G., Jackson, D., Wilkes, L. and Vickers, M. (2013) 'Personal resilience in nurses and midwives: Effects of a work-based educational intervention', *Contemporary Nurse: A Journal for the Australian Nursing Profession*, 45 (1): 134–43.

Mills, J., Wand, T. and Fraser, J.A. (2015) 'On self-compassion and self-care in nursing: Selfish or essential for compassionate care?', *International Journal of Nursing Studies*, 52, 791–3.

Neff, K. (2003) 'Self-compassion: An alternative conceptualization of a healthy attitude toward oneself', *Self and Identity*, 2: 85–101.

Neff, K. (2015) *Self-Compassion: Stop Beating Yourself Up and Leave Insecurity Behind.* London: Yellow Kite.

Neff, K. (2017) 'The chemicals of care: How self-compassion manifests in our bodies, self-compassion', Self-Compassion. Available at: http://self-compassion.org/the-chemicals-of-care-how-self-compassion-manifests-in-our-bodies/ (accessed October 2017).

NHS Digital (2017) NHS *Workforce Statistics: March 2017, Provisional Statistics.* Available at: www.content.digital.nhs.uk/catalogue/PUB24214 (accessed August 2017).

Nursing Midwifery Council (NMC) (2017) *Future Nurse Standards and Education Framework: Consultation.* Available at: www.nmc.org.uk/globalassets/sitedocuments/councilpapersanddocuments/council-2017/council-item-7-may-2017.pdf (accessed October 2017).

Paldanius, A. and Maatta, K. (2011) 'What are students views of (loving) caring in nursing education in Finland?', *International Journal of Caring Sciences*, 4 (2): 81–9.

Point of Care Foundation (2017) *Schwartz Rounds*. Available at: www.pointofcarefoundation. org.uk/our-work/schwartz-rounds (accessed 24 April 2017).

Robichaud, A.L. (2003) 'Healing and feeling: The clinical ontology of emotion', *Bioethics*, 17 (1): 59–68.

Royal College of Nursing (RCN) (2017) *RCN Guidance for Mentors of Nursing and Midwifery Students*. Available at: www.rcn.org.uk/-/media/royal-college-of-nursing/documents/publica tions/2017/may/pub-006133.pdf (accessed July 2017).

Sangharakshita, B. (1990) *A Guide to the Buddhist Path*. London: Windhorse, p. 93.

Senyuva, E., Kaya, H., Isik, B. and Bodur, G. (2014) 'Relationship between self-compassion and emotional intelligence in nursing students', *International Journal of Nursing Practice*, 20: 588–96.

Sturm, B. and Dellert, J. (2016) 'Exploring nurses' personal dignity, global self-esteem and work satisfaction', *Nursing Ethics*, 23 (4): 384–400.

Versterinen, S., Suhonen, M., Isola, A. and Paasivaara, L. (2012) 'Nurse managers' leadership styles in Finland', *Nursing Research and Practice*. Available at: http://dx.doi. org/10.1155/2012/605379 (accessed October 2017).

Waddington, K. (2016) 'The compassion gap in UK universities', *International Practice Development Journal*, 6 (1): 5.

Wilkin, S. (1846) *The Works of Sir Thomas Browne*, Vol. 2. London: Henry G. Bohn.

8

Collaborative Working

Mary Kennedy

Alone we can do so little; together we can do so much. (Helen Keller, Lash, (1980: 489), American writer and social activist, 1880–1968)

Chapter aims

- Partnership working and collaboration.
- Partnership working in the context of nursing practice.
- The role of interprofessional education (IPE).
- Working in partnership with patients and families.

Introduction

In today's National Health Service (NHS), there is an expectation that health professionals will work in a collaborative, integrated way to deliver safe, effective, person-centred care. This is not a new concept and there are many references to the need for different professional groups to work together in partnership and in collaboration (Department of Health, DH, 2015; NHS England, 2014). Enabling patients and families to be active participants in their health and healthcare is a fundamental goal and is well established in health policy and healthcare guidelines. An example of this is the *Five Year Forward View*, where partnership working is highlighted, providing examples of service developments created in partnership with patients and communities (NHS England, 2014).

The NHS is an integrated system of organisations and services, and is bound together by the principles and values reflected in the NHS Constitution (DH, 2015). The Constitution gives a commitment to working in partnership with other organisations in the interests of patients, local communities and the wider population (ibid.). It pledges to patients that NHS staff will 'work in partnership with you, your family, carers and representatives', and informs them that they have the right to be involved in planning and making decisions about their healthcare with the relevant information and support provided (ibid.: 10).

In nursing, partnership working with patients and their families is a key priority to ensure the delivery of care that is person-centred, safe and effective (Nursing and Midwifery Council, NMC, 2015). This is clearly outlined in the NMC Code of Professional Standards (ibid.), which states that registered nurses are required to: 'Prioritise people', and to listen and respond to their preferences and concerns.

With increasing demands and growing financial pressures, there has never been a greater need for the NHS to make a concentrated effort to get partnership working right. However, some may say that 'partnership working' has long been a catchphrase with very little evidence of collaboration to support it. The commitment of the Department of Health to putting patients at the centre of healthcare was evident in its report Patients First and Foremost (DH, 2013b) published in response to the Francis Inquiry (2013) and failures of care at the Mid Staffordshire NHS Trust. If the NHS is to achieve this aim, and survive and thrive, then it needs to work more collaboratively in order to share its collective strengths as partners across the entire system.

Partnership and collaboration

Although the terms 'partnership' and 'collaboration' are rarely specifically defined, in most understandings successful partnerships rely on good systems of interprofessional collaboration (Lymbery, 2006). In healthcare, the term 'partnership' is often used in relation to interprofessional working or collaborations between different organisations and has been defined by the World Health Organization (WHO) as occurring when:

> multiple health workers from different professional backgrounds provide comprehensive services by working with patients, their families, carers and communities to deliver the highest quality of care across settings. (2010: 13)

As highlighted earlier, the idea of partnership working is not a new concept. Dickinson (2007) suggests that to some extent, it is a necessary mechanism to overcome some of the structural difficulties associated with the existence of separate health and social care systems. For this reason, she regards partnership as an important concept, endeavouring to bridge the complexities caused by boundaries in terms of policy, practice and for services users (ibid.).

Whatever definition is applied, it is clear that in order for care to be enabling, there should be a partnership between healthcare professionals and patients (The Health Foundation, 2014), working together so as to understand what is important to the person, making decisions about their care and treatment, and identifying and achieving their goals (WHO, 2010; NHS England, 2014; The Health Foundation, 2014; DH, 2015; NMC, 2015).

What are the benefits of partnership and collaboration?

Given the way that today's health and social care is provided, it is even more dependent on partnership working, promoting a strong commitment to developing effective teams that can work together across organisational boundaries and across different professional groups. Collaboration is about moving away from individual ways of working and moving instead towards developing effective teams, particularly for those on the frontline.

Equally, as concerns for quality of care continue to grow, the need for collaborative practice is increasingly of high priority, thereby making a compelling argument for different professional groups to be building partnerships and collaborative ways of working – and not in individual silos! There is a convincing evidence to support that team-working improves patient care and that collaborative practice by healthcare professionals strengthens health systems, patient satisfaction, acceptance of care and improved patient outcomes (WHO, 2010). However, even though there is evidence that organisational and health professionals understand and appreciate the need for interprofessional collaboration, for some reason this doesn't always transfer into practice (Towle, 2016). Why is this? What are the possible barriers?

Following a review of the literature on professional 'silos' and 'effective interprofessional teams', Towle (ibid.) identified that between 2011 and 2016, there were over 9000 articles published documenting how and why nurses need to work collaboratively within interprofessional teams. She also highlighted that over decades, articles, reports and other evidence-based research had clearly established that working collaboratively within interprofessional teams was not only essential but also critical in the delivery of quality, safe, patient-centred care (ibid.).

Since the publication of key inquiries into failures of care in NHS hospitals (Francis, 2013; Berwick, 2013), there is now a greater awareness that the NHS needs to change if it is to continue to deliver safe, high-quality, sustainable care. To achieve this, it needs to be equipped with a workforce that can enable this to happen and be able to meet a variety of challenges: an ageing population; greater migration; inequalities; and providing better support for those living with complex health and social care needs (Mulvale et al., 2016; NHS England, 2014). Ultimately, if different professional groups are to work more efficiently and effectively to address these issues, then interprofessional collaborative practice has a key role to play.

How does this relate to nursing practice?

We are all acutely aware that the NHS is facing turbulent times, with financial constraints, complex care environments and demands for services that are continuously straining capacity and that will only continue to do so. For nurses, who spend more time with patients than any other clinical group, this can be challenging. Although it places them in an ideal position to promote patient participation, there is also an expectation that they will meet the efficiency targets of their organisation, often with limited resources and low staffing levels. This may go some way towards explaining why nurses, along with various other healthcare professionals, are inclined to work in professional 'silos' (Towle, 2016).

The notion of professional 'silos' tends to create debate. For example, Towle (ibid.) poses the question on whether health profession students are graduating without the critical skills required to work effectively and efficiently within interprofessional teams. One way of addressing this is through interprofessional education (IPE). This has resulted in the publication of guidelines such as Interprofessional Education Guidelines from the Centre for the Advancement of Interprofessional Education (CAIPE) (Barr et al., 2017). Evidence suggests that adverse events can occur as a result of poor collaboration and communication, and public inquiries into failures in healthcare have strengthened the argument for more collaborative approaches (Francis, 2013; Berwick 2013). As a result, more nursing programmes now include IPE content in their curricula. For example, in the UK, the Nursing and Midwifery Council's Quality Assurance Framework (2017) requires that approved education institutions must evidence that they have an interprofessional learning policy and processes for this in place, including simulation suites that support interprofessional learning and assessment opportunities.

Interprofessional education (IPE)

The CAIPE guidelines developed by Barr, Ford & Gray et al (2017: 14) recognise IPE as occurring when 'members or students of two or more professions learn with, from and about each other to improve collaboration and the quality of care and services'. The aim of CAIPE is to promote and develop IPE in collaboration with like-minded organisations, both in the UK and abroad, for the benefit of patients and clients. It suggests that IPE can impact through:

- Improving working relations amongst health professions.
- Modifying negative attitudes and perceptions.
- Coping with needs that exceed the capacity of one profession.
- Enhancing job satisfaction and easing stress.
- Increasing workforce flexibility.
- Integrating specialist and holistic care.

The WHO (2010) recognised that IPE offers the potential to create a collaborative workforce, facilitating collaborative practice and enabling best health outcomes for local populations. This view is also supported in the UK's healthcare policy, with the integration of health and social care, a focus on patient safety and person-centred care (NHS England, 2014; Health Foundation, 2014; DH, 2015; NMC, 2015).

To ensure the health and safety of the public, health professionals employed in the NHS are legally required to be registered with their professional regulatory body. In the UK, the Nursing and Midwifery Council (NMC) is the regulator for nursing and midwifery, and sets and reviews standards for education, training, conduct and performance in its profession. In common with other professions, nursing has its own standards for competence, which every nurse must maintain throughout their career in order to remain on the register (NMC, 2015). The four domains where nurses are required to demonstrate competencies are:

1. Professional values
2. Communication and interpersonal skills
3. Nursing practice and decision-making
4. Leadership, management and team-working

The Code states that:

> There is a clear expectation throughout the competency framework that nurses will engage in partnership working and must
>
> - Build partnerships and therapeutic relationships through safe, effective and nondiscriminatory communication. They must take account of individual differences, capabilities and needs.
> - Work in partnership with service users, carers, groups, communities and organisations … They must manage risk, and promote health and well-being while aiming to empower choices that promote self-care and safety.
> - Promote selfcare and management whenever possible, helping people to make choices about their healthcare needs, involving families and carers where appropriate, to maximize their ability to care for themselves. (NMC, 2010: 6, 8–9

Equivalent interprofessional competency frameworks to those outlined by the NMC (2015) have also emerged from America and Canada, using similar terminologies. In America, the Interprofessional Education Collaborative (IPEC) established four core competency domains as a structure for IPE (IPEC, 2011. Similarly, the Canadian Interprofessional Health Collaborative (CIHC) established six competency domains for their National Interprofessional Competency Framework (2010).

As shown in Table 8.1, there are some common threads across the competencies, demonstrating a cross-professional consensus on the implementation and value of interprofessional teamwork and collaboration.

Interestingly, some of the challenges to interprofessional education over the last five decades are recurring themes, including curricular limitations and professional role issues (Lewitt et al 2015). Each profession is bound by its own roles, skills and responsibilities. However, this doesn't mean that they should work in isolation with patients and their families – their professional 'silos' – without collaborating with other health and social care professionals who are involved in the care pathway and make up the multiprofessional team.

You may find it helpful to reflect on 'role and responsibilities' and ask, 'What matters to you?' Sometimes, it's worth stepping back and reflecting on our individual roles – what we do and how we do it – and, most importantly, whether what we're doing is what the patient wants. In Chapter 3, Martin and Harrison (2017) raise an interesting question, 'Is nursing a service with (too) many masters?',

Table 8.1 Competency Frameworks

NMC (2015)	IPEC (2011)	CIHC (2010)
1. Professional values	1. Values and ethics	1. Role clarification
2. Communication and interpersonal skills	2. Roles and responsibilities	2. Team functioning
		3. Patient/client/family/ community-centred care
3. Nursing practice and decision-making	3. Interprofessional communication	
4. Leadership, management and team-working	4. Teams and teamwork	4. Collaborative leadership
		5. Interprofessional communication
		6. Interprofessional conflict management

and provide a useful model of the many different people and services with whom nurse interacts on a daily basis. On the frontline, delivering 24-hour care, the nurse is often involved in various aspects of patient care and has many roles and responsibilities. Over her nursing career, the author has heard nurses referred to as 'jack of all trades, master of none'! It is this variety of knowledge and skills accumulated by nurses as they move through their careers that makes their contribution to patient care unique.

Understanding our own roles and responsibilities and those of other professionals is not always as simple as it may seem. With increased interprofessional collaboration, there is the potential for boundaries between professional roles and responsibilities to become blurred, leading to possible confusion as to which profession should implement a particular treatment or intervention. At times, this can lead to a problem of 'interprofessional conflict'.

Bainbridge et al. (2010) suggest that there are several reasons for conflict between professional groups, one being different professional groups not understanding one another's roles and accountability. They suggest that this is mainly because, throughout their training, different professional groups are socialised in diverse ways, learning different rules and ways of practicing unique to their specific professional training. Drinka and Clark (2000, cited in Reeves et al., 2017) proposed that this may be potentially resolved by understanding that other professionals have different perspectives of patient care and that the contribution of each of these perspectives should be equally valued.

Interestingly, although the IPEC only updated the current framework in 2016, it has already been suggested that further developments are required. Specifically, Dow et al. (2017) suggest that 'networking' should be added to the 'teams and teamwork' domain. They consider networking as an additional important conceptualisation for interprofessional practice as, 'rather than working in discrete teams, healthcare professionals often work in large, heterogeneous, and dynamic groups as well as networks' (Dow et al., 2017: 678). This is supported by Reeves et al. (2017), who suggest the inclusion of other forms of interprofessional work: 'interprofessional collaboration' and 'coordination'. They conclude by recommending further work and developments into future refinements of collaborative competence, and further developments are likely.

Partnership working with patients and families

In 2016, the King's Fund published a report on *Patients as Partners*, reinforcing the importance of collaborative relationship in healthcare (Seale, 2016). In the introduction to the report, they provide a clear statement of their belief that patients, carers, third sector and communities are central to the future NHS, and propose that these perspectives are essential as 'patients are why the NHS exists' (ibid.: 3). Again, this concept is not new, with much of healthcare policy being focused on integrating services and putting the patient at the centre of service delivery, research and education (NHS England, 2014; DH, 2015). As mentioned earlier the Department of Health echoed a similar view in its report Patients First and Foremost, which it published following the Francis Inquiry in 2013. Again, the WHO (2017) has argued that participation exercises patients' healthcare rights, enabling them to be partners in making healthcare decisions. Nevertheless, the concept of patient participation remains a complex issue, causing widespread debate.

Shared decision-making

Partnership working is closely associated with promoting choice and shared decision-making. Shared decision-making is basically a conversation based on partnership that brings the healthcare practitioner and patient together to choose healthcare options through exchanging information and evidence about their options, as well as discussing the patient's values so as to elicit his or her preferences (Groen-van de Ven et al., 2017).

What does shared decision-making look like in practice? And how can it be supported? Elwyn et al. (2017) describe a useful three-talk model of shared decision-making based on 'team talk', 'option talk' and 'decision talk', depicting a process of collaboration and deliberation (Figure 8.1). The three-talk model portrays conversational steps, initiated by providing support when introducing options, followed by strategies to compare and discuss trade-offs, before deliberation based on informed preferences.

In this sense, partnership working and shared decision-making are broadly associated with person-centred care, which has four key principles (Health Foundation, 2014):

1.   The person is treated with dignity, compassion and respect.
2.   Care is coordinated.

3. Care is personalised.

4. Care enables them to live an independent and fulfilling life.

For most nurses, partnership working is an ongoing process in day-to-day care delivery with patients and their families, and reference is made to partnership working and decision-making in the NMC core competencies: 'decision making must be shared with service users, carers, families and informed by critical analysis of a full range of possible interventions' (2015: 7). In this context, partnership working serves to enhance a patient's sense of empowerment, giving them some control over their own well-being and healthcare decisions.

Partnership working with service users, carers and families occurs in an interprofessional context and in many different situations. For example, nurses may work in partnership during local initiatives to improve care quality, and at a macro-level in co-designing new services.

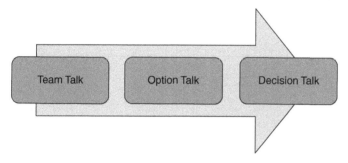

1. **Team Talk:** Work together, describe choices, offer support and ask about goals
2. **Option Talk:** Discuss alternatives using risk communication principles
3. **Decision Talk:** Get to informed preferences, make preferences based on decisions

Figure 8.1   Three-talk model of shared decision-making (adapted from Elwyn et al., 2017)

Promoting Participation

Through participating in the decision-making process, and taking part in treatment and service evaluation, patients can contribute to improvements in healthcare – from a patient-consumer perspective they are also able to demand quality services (Souliotis, 2016). This is recognised as part of the NHS England *Five Year Forward View* (2014), where Simon Stevens, NHS England's Chief Executive, commissioned a set of 'high impact actions' for accelerating the adoption of person and community-centred approaches to health and care. It supports the vision of a health and care system that fully engages people in their health, care and well-being, through working in partnership with communities and the voluntary sector (People and Communities Board, PCB, 2017: 5). This is captured in the following statement by the PCB:

A growing body of policy, evidence, thinking and practice is now pointing the NHS to work in these ways. The reason is that they improve health; improve the outcomes of care and treatment; improve the allocation of resources; and build social value and community resilience. Health and care professionals are increasingly finding that these approaches enable them to practice their disciplines in more humane, holistic and rewarding ways.

Models of participation

McKinnon (2013) offers the view that levels of participation underpin partnership working. One model of participation that has stood the test of time is Arnstein's (1969) 'Ladder of Participation' (cited in McKinnon, 2013) (Figure 8.2). In developing the model, Arnstein (1969) envisaged a ladder of ascent, from manipulation, through tokenistic steps, to full citizen power (Gibson et al., 2012). Traditionally, the model has been used to help health professionals identify and understand the

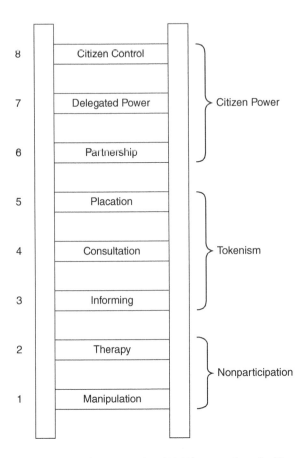

Figure 8.2 Arnstein's Ladder of Participation (1969), reproduced with permission of Taylor & Francis

power imbalance between themselves and their patients. In applying the model, vast differences in power – ranging from non-participation, tokenistic autonomy and full patient power – can be highlighted (McKinnon, 2013).

Despite it being many years since Arnstein's work first appeared, Gibson et al. (2012) believe that it constructively details the way in which participation in the process may often be little more than manipulation. As a result, they propose that the Ladder of Participation remains a useful first base when considering the broader conceptualisation of public involvement, highlighting the need for any discussions to be 'firmly based in an understanding of the central role of power' (Gibson et al., 2012: 535).

The eight stages of power represented by the Arnstein's Ladder can be usefully applied in health and social care settings. The two bottom rungs of the ladder, (1) *manipulation* and (2) *therapy*, are described as levels of 'non-participation', where the aim is to cure or educate patients towards changing themselves rather than giving them a say in decisions about their healthcare. Rungs three and four then progress to (3) *informing* and (4) *consultation*, described as 'tokenism' and are the first steps toward active participation. At this level, the health professional informs the patient of their rights and options within the care process and, therefore, by becoming more actively engaged, they have more of an opportunity for their voice to be heard. For example, through taking part in patient surveys or being involved in meetings or consultations. The fifth rung, (5) *placation*, also forms part of tokenism and, although at this level the patient is actively involved in planning their care, the ultimate decisions regarding their care or treatment are still made by the health professionals. The last three rungs of the ladder are described as 'Citizen Power' and include (6) *partnership*, (7) *delegated power* and (8) *citizen control*. This level of participation is reflected in the three-talk model described by Elwyn et al. (2017), where the planning and decision-making are shared and the power is redistributed via negotiation with the patient, their family and the healthcare professionals. At the 'Citizen Power' level, the patient has total control and power regarding their own healthcare.

Although Arnstein's Ladder is a useful model that has stood the test of time, Elwyn's three-talk model as depicted in Figure 8.1 is more relevant in today's healthcare environment and in supporting shared decision-making in practice. It also complements other, more current, partnership-based approaches such as 'Experience-Based Co-Design' (EBCD) (Robert et al., 2015). This is a form of Participatory Action Research (PAR) used in healthcare and refers to patients and carers working in partnership with health professionals to improve services. EBCD has been defined as: an approach that enables staff and patients (or other service users) to co-design services and/or care pathways, together in partnership' (Point of Care Foundation, 2018).

As described by Robert et al. (2015), EBCD is a six-stage process that usually takes 9–12 months to complete (Table 8.2). This is a fairly lengthy process and, given the current demands on services and the lack of health and human resources, this could be a barrier to implementation. However, as pointed out by Coulter et al. (2014), the NHS has been collecting data on patients' experience of care for more than a decade but few providers are systematically using the information to improve services. They argue that a national institute of 'user' experience should be created so as to draw the data together, determine how to interpret the results and put them

Table 8.2 EBCD six-stage process (adapted from Robert et al., 2015)

- Setting up the project

- Gathering staff experiences through observation and in-depth interviews

- Gathering patient and carer experiences through 12–15 filmed narrative-based interviews

- Bringing staff, patients and carers together to share their experiences of a service and identify their shared priorities for improvement, prompted by an edited 30 minute 'trigger' film of patient narratives

- Small groups of patients and staff work on the identified priorities (typically 4–6) over three or four months

- Celebration and review event

into practice (ibid.), as Robert et al. commented: 'Patients provide insight, wisdom, and ideas, and we urgently need to include them more creatively as partners in change' (2015: 2).

Conclusion

As highlighted throughout this chapter, in order for partnership working to be effective, health and social care professionals need to have well-developed interprofessional skills for working with patients, families and communities. By fully embracing partnership working and adopting collaborative approaches, different professional groups can be supported to establish trusting relationships that empower others and are based on common values and mutual respect. Personal reflection on the experience of partnership working, listening to the experiences of patients and families and collaborating with multiprofessional teams can help to support professional development and promote partnership working.

References

Arnstein, S.R. (1969) 'A ladder of citizen participation', *Journal of the American Planning Association*, 35: 216–24.
Bainbridge, P.T., Nasmith, L., Orchard, C. and Wood, V. (2010) 'Competencies for interprofessional collaboration', *Journal of Physical Therapy Education*, 24: 6–11.
Barr, H., Ford, J., Gray, R. et al. (2017) *Interprofessional Education Guidelines*. Fareham: Centre for Advancement of Interprofessional Education (CAIPE). Available at: www.caipe.org/resources/publications/caipe-publications/caipe-2017-interprofessional-education-guidelines-barr-h-ford-j-gray-r-helme-m-hutchings-m-low-h-machin-reeves-s (accessed January 2018).

Berwick, D. (2013) *A Promise to Learn: A Commitment to Act – Improving the Safety of Patients in England*. London: Department of Health.

Canadian Interprofessional Health Collaborative (CIHC) (2010) *A National Interprofessional Competency Framework*. Vancouver: CIHC.

Coulter, A., Locock, L., Ziebland, S. and Calabrese, J. (2014) *Collecting Data on Patient Experience is not Enough: They Must Be Used to Improve Care*. Available at: www.bmj.com/content/348/bmj.g2225 (accessed December 2017).

Department of Health (DH) (2013a) *Department of Health Commits to Reconnecting with Patients in Response to Francis Inquiry*. London: DH. Available at: www.gov.uk/government/news/department-of-health-commits-to-reconnecting-with-patients-in-response-to-francis-inquiry (accessed December 2017).

DH (2013b) *Patients first and foremost: The Initial Government Response to the Report of The Mid Staffordshire NHS Foundation Trust Public Inquiry*. Available at: https://assets.publishing.service.gov.uk/government/uploads/system/uploads/attachment_data/file/170701/Patients_First_and_foremost.pdf (accessed 24 April 2018).

DH (2015) *The NHS Constitution: The NHS Belongs to Us All*. London: DH. Available at: www.gov.uk/government/uploads/system/uploads/attachment_data/file/480482/NHS_Constitution_WEB.pdf (accessed December 2017).

Dickinson, H. (2007) 'Evaluating the outcomes of health and social care partnerships: The POET approach, *Research, Policy and Planning*, 25: 79–92.

Dow, A., Zhu, X., Sewell, D., Banas, C., Mishra, V. and Tu, S.-P. (2017) 'Teamwork on the rocks: Rethinking interprofessional practice as networking', *Journal of Interprofessional Care*, 31 (6): 677–8. Available at: https://doi.org/10.1080/13561820.2017.13440489 (accessed November 2017).

Elwyn, G., Durand, M.A., Song, J. et al. (2017) 'A three-talk model for shared decision making: Multistage consultation process', *BMJ 359*: j4891. Available at: www.bmj.com/content/359/bmj.j4891 (accessed November 2017).

Francis, R. (2013) *Report of the Mid Staffordshire NHS Foundation Trust Public Inquiry*. London: The Stationery Office.

Gibson, A., Britten, N. and Lynch, J. (2012) 'Theoretical directions for an emancipatory concept of patient and public involvement', *Health: An Interdisciplinary Journal for the Social Study of Health, Illness and Medicine*, 16 (5): 531–47. Available at: http://journals.sagepub.com/doi/pdf/10.1177/1363459312438563 (accessed December 2017).

Groen-van de Ven, L., Smits, C., Graaff, F. et al. (2017) 'Involvement of people with dementia in making decisions about their lives: A qualitative study that appraises shared decision-making concerning daycare', *BMJ Open*, 7: 1–13.

The Health Foundation (2014) *Person-Centred Care Made Simple: What Everyone Should Know about Person-Centred Care*. Available at: www.health.org.uk/sites/health/files/PersonCentredCareMadeSimple.pdf (accessed December 2017).

Interprofessional Education Collaborative Expert Panel (2011) *Core Competencies for Interprofessional Collaborative Practice: Report of an Expert Panel*. Washington, DC: Association for American Medical Colleges.

Lash, J.P. (1980) *Helen and Teacher: The Story of Helen Keller and Anne Sullivan Macy*. New York: Delacorte Press/Seymour Lawrence.

Lewitt, S.M., Cross, B., Sheward, L. and Beirne, P. (2015) *Interprofessional Education to Support Collaborative Practice: An Interdisciplinary Approach, Society for Research into Higher Education*. Hamilton: University of West Scotland.

Lymbery, M. (2006) 'United we stand? Partnership working in health and social care and the role of social work in services for older people', *British Journal of Social Work*, 36: 1119–34.

McKinnon, J. (2013) 'The case for concordance: Value and application in nursing practice', *British Journal of Nursing*, 22: 766–71.

Mulvale, G., Embrett, M. and Donya Razavi, S. (2016) '"Gearing Up" to improve interprofessional collaboration in primary care: A systematic review and conceptual framework', *BMC Family Practice*, 17: 83.

NHS England (2014) *Five Year Forward View*. London: NHS England. Available at: www.england.nhs.uk/wp-content/uploads/2014/10/5yfv-web.pdf (accessed December 2017).

Nursing and Midwifery Council (NMC) (2010) *Standards for Competence for Registered Nurses*. London: NMC.

Nursing and Midwifery Council (NMC) (2015) *The NMC Code of Professional Standards*. London: NMC.

NMC (2017) *Quality Assurance Framework for Nursing and Midwifery Education*. London: NMC. Available at: www.nmc.org.uk/education/quality-assurance-of-education/qa-framework-for-education/ (accessed November 2017).

People and Communities Board (PCB) (2017) *A New Relationship with People and Communities: Actions for Delivering Chapter 2 of the NHS Five Year Forward View*. London: King's Fund.

Point of Care Foundation (2018) Available at: www.pointofcarefoundation.org.uk (accessed 12 March 2018).

Reeves, S., Palaganas, J. and Zierler, B. (2017) 'Teamwork, collaboration, coordination, and networking: Why we need to distinguish between different types of interprofessional practice', *Journal of Interprofessional Care*, 32: 1–3.

Robert, G., Cornwell, J., Locock, L. et al. (2015) 'Patients and staff as co-designers of healthcare Services', *BMJ*, 350: g7714.

Seale, B. (2016) *Patients as Partners: Building Collaborative Relationships among Professionals, Patients, Carers and Communities*. London: King's Fund.

Souliotis, K. (2016) 'Patient participation in contemporary health care: Promoting a versatile patient role', *Health Expectations*, 19: 175–8.

Towle, A. (2016) 'Nurses must knock down professional "silos" and create quality, safe and effective interprofessional teams, from the inside looking out: A healthcare providers experience being the family member', *Journal of Nursing and Care*, 5: 3.

World Health Organization (WHO) (2010) *Framework for Action on Interprofessional Education and Collaborative Practice*. Geneva: WHO. Available at: http://apps.who.int/iris/bitstream/10665/70185/1/WHO_HRH_HPN_10.3_eng.pdf?ua=1 (accessed December 2017).

WHO (2017) *Human Rights and Health*. Geneva: WHO. Available at: www.who.int/mediacentre/factsheets/fs323/en/ (accessed December 2017).

9

Mental Parkour

Freeing the Mind

Martin Harrison and Peter J. Martin

When we are no longer able to change a situation, we are challenged to change ourselves. (Frankl, 2006 [1946]: 112)

Chapter aims

- See the world from a different perspective.
- Enhance and develop creative thinking and problem-solving.
- Learn to improve our positive risk-taking in everyday practice.

Introduction

If we were able to talk to Florence Nightingale while she was working at a military hospital in Scutari in the 1850s, Dr Will Pooley, MBE, nursing people with Ebola in Sierra Leone, or Staff Nurse Smith working today in an Intensive Care Unit in a Manchester hospital, all would describe health and healthcare as dynamic, in a constant state of change.

Unfortunately, it is all too easy to look at the world in which we work as static: we go to work and we come home. It can be summed up in that commonly used phrase: 'It's just the same old, same old.' But the UK health system is far from static. It is constantly facing new challenges, for example:

- The economic climate.
- The political climate, e.g. the UK–EU relationship.
- Demographic changes, e.g. an ageing population.

- Medical and pharmaceutical advances in treatments.
- Changes in the philosophical approach to healthcare.
- Increased technology and the ubiquity of health information on the Internet.

These challenges require the health and social care system to evolve as the rapid pace of this change is likely to continue for the foreseeable future. For health and social care staff, it means that we must adjust to this change: some will achieve this effectively and some will do so less effectively. We need to learn how to work within this dynamic environment in a way that enables us to deliver the best quality nursing care that we are able to deliver, whilst not being harmed in the process.

Managing change can be stressful and the more stressed we become, the more difficult it is to *look over the parapet* at the wider world in which we exist; because, in doing so, we may find more things that challenge our uncomfortable but safe world. Over the parapet might be another service reorganisation, a new audit form to complete or a new IT system to learn. We need to find some way of looking at the world, over the parapet, and of seeing it as a challenging place, but a challenge to be met rather than one that we perceive as impossibly overwhelming.

In this chapter, we use the analogy of 'parkour', or 'free-running', as a way of thinking creatively about how we continue to deliver health and social care in a contemporary care system, whilst paying attention to our own bio-psycho-socio-spiritual well-being. Sport England's *Active Lives Adult Survey* indicates that 101,800 parkour practitioners (aged 16+) had engaged in the sport at least twice in the preceding 28 days (2017). Parkour UK (2017) offers the following definition:

> Parkour/Freerunning/Art du Deplacement is the non-competitive physical discipline of training to move freely over and through any terrain using only the abilities of the body, principally through running, jumping, climbing and quadrupedal movement. In practice it focuses on developing the fundamental attributes required for such movement, which include functional strength and fitness, balance, spatial awareness, agility, coordination, precision, control and creative vision.

In this chapter, the analogy of Parkour is not presented as an *evidence-based tool*, but simply as a way of helping to stimulate creative thinking about the health and social care environments in which we work. For example, if we go to our local park, we might notice the trees, the flower beds, the ducks on the pond. We might pause and rest against the railing around the pond while we watch people whiling away a sunny afternoon. But through the eyes of a parkour practitioner, this same scene may look very different:

> you can practice it [Parkour] anywhere (natural or manmade), as long as there are obstacles to interact with. … Even though spots that are dense with obstacles are usually considered better, limiting yourself to a single obstacle or 'bad' spots can be just as beneficial … the true spirit of Parkour is to adapt to the obstacles at hand. Even a simple rail can provide plenty of opportunities for practice. (Ford, 2017)

If a parkour practitioner sees the world differently, how might she or he see the world in which *you* work?

The view from here?

In this section, we want to examine ways in which we can encourage ourselves to look at the world from a different perspective: how we can break out of predictable ways of thinking. Mezirow and Associates suggested that we 'make meaning' through our unique 'meaning schemes' and 'meaning perspectives' (1990: 2). A 'meaning scheme' is the way in which you express your views to the world, whilst a 'meaning perspective' is your view of the world that underpins the 'meaning scheme'. For example, think about the NHS in the UK and how you regard this organisation? In Table 9.1, you will see viewpoint (a) and viewpoint (b); whilst you may not wholly subscribe to one view or the other, you may feel more drawn to (a) or to (b).

Table 9.1   Meaning Schemes

Meaning Schemes (What we express daily to the world)	
(a) One view	**(b) An alternative view**
• Our budget is never sufficient to meet our needs	• We could always do with more money to improve our services, but we deliver the best service we can within the budget we have
• The targets that are set for us are never achievable	• Targets are important as they help us learn from others how to improve our service
• We are always short of staff	• The 'right' staffing in healthcare service is problematic; currently, there are definitely deficits
• We just focus on getting through the shift	• Getting through the day is important but we need to plan for the future also
• Everyone's leaving, they've had enough	• Working in healthcare has always been stressful; that isn't going to change, so we need to work out how we can build resilience in all our staff so they don't get damaged

Mezirow and Associates (ibid.) argue that underpinning these meaning perspectives are robust meaning schemes. In Table 9.2, you will find the meaning schemes that accompany the meaning perspectives in Table 9.1. Looking at column (a) in the two tables, you should see that Table 9.2 is the overarching view that is verbalised through statements in Table 9.1. The same applies to the (b) columns.

Table 9.2   Meaning Perspectives

Meaning Perspectives (Thinking that underlies our meaning schemes)	
(a) One view	**(b) An alternative view**
The NHS is an overburdened organisation, run by burnt-out staff, operating in a country that doesn't care about the health of its population	The NHS is a unique sociopolitical achievement that represents a high point in a civilised society

....

Activity 9.1   Reflective Exercise – Mental Parkour

On our way to work, we may navigate through the city using pavements, junctions and pedestrian crossings. As we engage with the environment in a particular (traditional) way, simultaneously, a parkour practitioner might be:

> Jumping over bollards, climbing up walls or rolling over concrete roofs; these spectacular movements show what the human body is capable of – but they also highlight how the city can be navigated in very different ways. (Mould, 2017)
> Look again at Table 9.1 and Table 9.2. Which side did you most closely relate to: (a) or (b)?

- Now metaphorically take a *leap off one parapet* onto a neighboring one. Move your thinking from one side of Table 9.2 to the other. It will be uncomfortable.
- Pause and find your point of balance.
- You should now have shifted your perspective from one side of Table 9.2 to the other.

Now, metaphorically look around you. Then, taking your time and thinking carefully about being in a different 'pair of shoes' to those that you normally wear, ask yourself the following questions:

- How would it feel to come to work every day with this underpinning attitude?
- Can you recall working with anyone who seemed to hold this perspective?
- How might everyday events in your workplace look different?
- How might you seem different to your colleagues?
- How might you view your colleagues differently?

You are now free to leap back onto the parapet on which you feel most comfortable. You can do this because you can legitimately say that you have looked at the world from a different perspective.

....

Being realistic: What can and can't be changed by one person

Simply thinking about our assumptions will not, in itself, dramatically increase funding for the NHS or locate thousands more nurses just looking for the opportunity to work in the NHS. In a publicly funded service such as the NHS, the power to effect fundamental changes within it is part of the national economy, and making poor/good decisions lies with our elected politicians and appointed senior managers.

However, that is not the purpose of this chapter. This chapter is about you as an individual practitioner and how you cope daily with this dynamic environment. Shifting our perspective around throughout the day will help us to understand and manage some of the stresses and complexities that occur every day at work. For example, a ward that is short of staff will still be a ward that is short of staff, but shifting our perspective can help us focus on today rather than yesterday or tomorrow. An angry relative will still be an angry relative, but shifting our perspective can help us see things from their perspective, which will help us to retain our professionalism in a difficult situation. Challenging assumptions can help you take a more balanced view of the everyday 'impossible' situations with which we are confronted.

At this point, you may be thinking that you don't have the time to get all the work done on the shift, let alone have the time to worry about 'leaping off parapets' in order to take a different view. We offer this approach to *thinking differently* because, without the ability to look at the world differently, we can become increasingly constrained by a single view of the world. That view might be the (a) column in Tables 9.1 and 9.2, a view characterised by a disempowered person who doesn't feel listened to or cared about.

If this negative and demoralised perspective is shared by a staff group, then doing a job that requires compassion and the continuing management of intense emotional labour is going to be a problem. Consequently, the patients' experience is not likely to be positive. From here, it is but a very short step to a serious decline in standards (Francis, 2013). Francis (ibid.: 65–6) concluded that the most negative aspects of the culture at the Trust were:

- A lack of openness to criticism
- A lack of consideration for patients
- Defensiveness
- Looking inwards not outwards
- Secrecy
- Misplaced assumptions about the judgements and actions of others
- An acceptance of poor standards
- A failure to put the patient first in everything that is done

Not being complacent

Spending time thinking about the view we take of the world is important in more subtle ways. Our perspective might be that what occurred at Mid Staffs as reported in the Francis Report (2013) was unique, so unique that it could never happen 'here'. Such complacent thinking needs to be challenged in order to avoid replicating the failings, which were identified through the Francis Report, within our own services.

Francis (ibid.) reported on systemic problems and deficiencies in the very factors that should have prevented deterioration. It is important, therefore, not to demonise individuals for the overarching failures – many people throughout the organisation were responsible. But we should not forget that this gross failure comprised of many, many individual instances of poor practice:

23. The first inquiry heard harrowing personal stories from patients and patients' families about the appalling care received at the Trust. On many occasions, the accounts received related to basic elements of care and the quality of the patient experience. These included cases where:

- Patients were left in excrement in soiled bed clothes for lengthy periods;
- Assistance was not provided with feeding for patients who could not eat without help;
- Water was left out of reach;
- In spite of persistent requests for help, patients were not assisted in their toileting;
- Wards and toilet facilities were left in a filthy condition;
- Privacy and dignity, even in death, were denied;
- Triage in A&E was undertaken by untrained staff;
- Staff treated patients and those close to them with what appeared to be callous indifference. (Ibid.: 13)

Activity 9.2   Reflective Exercise

Spend a few moments thinking about your own ward or service when you were last in work. Take this day as a snapshot. You should focus on your own personal view rather than existing measures used in your workplace:

- On a rating scale of 1–10, how would you rate the quality of your own ward/service overall?
- What sort of measures would you consider important to rate separately and why are these factors particularly important, e.g. atmosphere, cleanliness, communication?
- How would you rate each of these individually?

Now, think about how many times, whilst you were answering these questions, you found yourself saying, 'Yes, that is only a "5", but …'
For example:

- The atmosphere is always a bit frantic *but* that's because two of the team are off sick and we can't get cover.
- One of the toilet cubicles is broken *but* the Estates Department are waiting for a new latch.

Whether there are pragmatic reasons for why your workplace is not as good as you would like it to be, we should always try and see it from another perspective. Remaining vigilant requires us to keep looking *over the parapet*, sometimes from an entirely new parapet, in order to adopt a different view of a single problem (Figure 9.1).

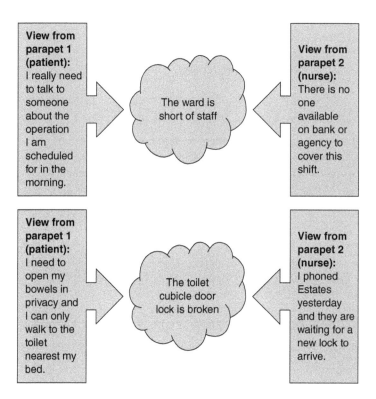

Figure 9.1 Same problem, different parapets

In order to help avoid an automatic, 'Yes, but…,' the work of Casement (1985) and Brookfield (1995) may be useful here. Patrick Casement worked as a psychoanalyst and wrote the influential work, *On Learning from the Patient* (1985). In this book, Casement explained how he was continually surprised by the patients whom he treated and how such 'surprise' offered new insights into his work. Casement coined the term the 'Internal Supervisor' (ibid.: 29) to describe the way in which he balanced his own view of an encounter with a patient alongside those of an 'imaginary' supervisor in order to get a clearer view of what was occurring.

Activity 9.3   Reflective Exercise

The following is a basic interpretation of how the Internal Supervisor might be experienced in a work-related context. A distressed relative is speaking to you, expressing concern about their partner's state of health. In your professional role, you may consider knowledge of:

- The patient.
- The condition experienced by the patient.

(Continued)

(Continued)

- Concerns about the patient's current state of health.
- Recent medical reports, tests, etc. received.
- The care plan.

More general awareness of:

- The relationship between the patient and partner.
- The partner's understanding of the health condition.
- Current workload and time available to spend with their partner.

Simultaneously, Casement suggests that the Internal Supervisor will be thinking:

- What is the underlying message that the partner is giving me (fear, anger, exhaustion, anxiety, etc.)?
- How am I responding to the partner?
- What words am I using in my response (jargon-free, honest, etc.)?
- How am I saying it (tone, volume, sensitivity, etc.)?
- What kind of person am I presenting to this person (rigid, professional, uncaring, compassionate, etc.)?

· ·

Brookfield (1995) suggests that we should use different 'lenses' so as to look critically at what we are doing (Figure 9.2). When you are next carrying out a part of your role (e.g., a wound dressing, de-escalation, delivering bad news, duty rota), stand in the shoes of others and look at yourself from these four perspectives.

In Activity 9.3 , Brookfield (ibid.) suggests that we should consider:

- What assumption do I hold about this encounter? For example:
  o I think that this person needs reassurance that their partner is receiving the best care that we can offer.
  o There is nothing more we can do at this point.

- What is the patient's partner view of this encounter? For example:
  o This nurse needs to tell me what is happening to my partner.
  o It needs to be in a way that I can understand.
  o We need to be doing something to help him.

- What are my colleagues' views about this encounter? For example:
  o [John] looks like he could do with a bit of help, the partner is becoming more, not less, distressed.

- What information can I draw from to help with this encounter from research, good practice, policies, etc.? For example:
  o Policies on communicating bad news.
  o Kubler-Ross's (1969) stages of grief, etc.

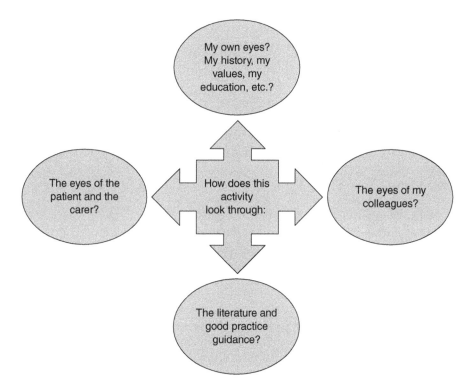

Figure 9.2 Brookfield's lenses (after Brookfield, 1995)

As you can see from Activity 9.3, John is trying to offer support to the partner based on his assumption about what is required, but hasn't fully appreciated the partner's perspective. The 'temperature' of such a conversation is only likely to rise as the two opposing perspectives clash.

Taking positive risks

It is interesting to consider why most of us chose not to behave in the same way as a skilled parkour practitioner. If we ask ourselves why, our answer would probably have, 'We don't want to get hurt!', somewhere in it. 'If I don't throw myself in the air, I won't get hurt' expresses something markedly similar to 'If I do my job exactly as I have been doing it for the past five years, I won't have anything to worry about,' or even, 'If I do my job exactly as I been told, I won't need to think about it.'

We need to look at how we manage risk. A parkour practitioner is only going to move creatively within an environment when she/he has fully embraced the risks associated with the next move. But no move is risk free and risk-taking occurs at the intersection of a person's own self-awareness and their reading of the terrain ahead.

In health and social care environments, there are additional levels of complexity but, regardless of this, Morgan argues that: 'It is not a matter of whether we take risks or not, it is a matter of how we take risks, and the process we use in coming to our conclusions' (2010b: 16, own emphasis).

....

Activity 9.4   Reflective Exercise

What are the positive risks in your service? Spend a few moments thinking about your workplace and try to identify examples of positive risk-taking. These can be small or large examples.
  Now, identify:

- What the actual risk is that is being managed.
- What processes have been put in place for its management.
- How agreement was reached that this was an acceptable risk.

....

Morgan (2010a: 21) offers a list of factors, which, he argues, will lead to confident, positive risk-taking. Many of these factors are not commonplace in health and social care services and, in consequence, defensive risk-taking is, perhaps, more customary. Confident, positive risk-taking, according to Morgan , is supported by:

- a person-centred approach with an in-depth focus on developing an assessment of strengths alongside problems and risks
- consensus across the team (and wider network of support) to think and work in this way
- appropriate tools to support the process of individual and team decision-making
- high-quality supervision and support
- priorities and resources focused on the creative challenge of doing things differently
- good team-based systems for recording and monitoring decisions
- clear ideas about what constitutes personal and collective responsibilities and accountability
- it becoming part of the fabric of training and service monitoring
- an organisation culture that understands and supports the philosophy and principles of good practice. (Morgan, 2010a: 21)

The avoidance of risk-taking is a natural defensive strategy that is exacerbated in stressed organisations and amongst stressed staff. However, Boardman and Roberts argue that we should be building in positive risk-taking in all services:

It needs to be understood that over-defensive, risk avoidant practice is bad practice and is associated with avoidable harm to both people who use services and practitioners. (2014: 3)

Boardman and Roberts, with reference to the UK Department of Health's *Independence, Choice and Risk: A Guide to Best Practice in Supported Decision Making*, indicate that the key legal and governance frameworks underpinning approaches to risk are:

1. *Duty of care*: Organisations must maintain an appropriate standard of care in their work and not be negligent. Individuals, who have a mental capacity to make a decision and choose voluntarily to live within a level of risk, are entitled to do so. In this case the law considers the person to have consented to the risk and there is thus no breach of duty of care and the organisation or individual cannot be considered negligent.

2. *Human rights* All public authorities and bodies have a duty not to act incompatibly with the European Convention of Human Rights. A balance needs to be struck between risk and the preservation of rights, especially when the person has capacity.

3. *Health and safety*: There is a legal duty on all employers to ensure, as far as reasonably practicable, the health, safety and welfare of their employees as well as the health and safety of those who use services. Health and Safety legislation should not block reasonable activity.

4. *Mental capacity*: This is concerned with a person's ability to make decisions for themselves and the principle enshrined in the Mental Capacity Act, 2005 is that they must be assumed to have capacity unless it is established that they do not. People with capacity may make unwise decisions. For those who lack capacity, decisions made on their behalf must be made in their best interests and with the least restriction.

5. *Fluctuating mental states and dementia*: The choices and wishes of people with fluctuating mental states and dementia must be respected and their risk agreements monitored and reviewed regularly. In these circumstances it is important to engage with families and carers.

6. *Safeguarding*: For people who are considered to be vulnerable there is a need to consider the factors of empowerment and safety, choice and risk. Practitioners need to consider when the need for protection overrides decision to promote choice and empowerment. (Boardman and Roberts, 2014: 6)

(Reproduced with permission of the Centre for Mental Health and the NHS Confederation Network.)

. . . .

Activity 9.5   Reflective Exercise

What other positive risks could be taken in your service? Spend a few moments thinking about your workplace and try to identify new areas where positive risk-taking could be considered. Again, these can be small or large examples. Now, identify:

(Continued)

(Continued)

- What is the actual risk that could be managed?
- If positive risk-taking were to be introduced, what would be the benefits for:
  - Patients
  - Staff
  - Organisation
- What processes would you need to put in place in order to establish a positive risk-taking strategy?
- How could agreement be reached that this was an acceptable risk.

. . . .

This section has been strongly influenced by positive risk-taking literature from mental health and social care services. We argue that it is just as relevant to acute physical care. As the quote from the NHS Commissioning Board states:

More of the same traditional relationship between providers of health and care services and passive recipient patients or service users won't be enough. Provider approaches will have to evolve towards making the empowerment, education and support of patients to self-manage their care a high and ongoing priority. (2015: 11)

There is increasing focus on empowering people to take more responsibility for their own health and social care needs. This is particularly notable, for example, in recovery (in mental health), personalised budgets, self-management and the idea of the 'expert patient' in long-term conditions. Telling people that they are responsible for their health will be limited in its impact if people do not first feel empowered to take decisions about their own lives: The possibility of risk is an inevitable consequence of empowered people taking decision about their own lives. (DH, 2007: 8)

Fluid movement

Parkour brings a sense of freedom of expression, challenge to social behaviour and autonomy that is inherently political. Perceptions of the way society works, how we view ourselves and those around us, as well as time and space, are all challenged by practicing Parkour. I see Parkour not as an apolitical activity but in fact as a potentially revolutionary one. The physical body becomes less constrained by societal views through the practice of Parkour. (Brown, 2017)

We would like to pose a conundrum between the two following statements:

1. Creating freedom in relation to how we view our world is liberating. From new perspectives come new ways of doing our job, new ways of engaging with people and new ways of thinking about problems.

2.   Creating freedom in relation to how we view our world is terrifying. From such new perspectives come challenges to the established hegemony. Those currently with power in the system do not welcome challenges and will respond with authority.

Both arguments are true and both have consequences, some of which will be unforeseeable. If even the thought of looking at your ward or service differently is too disturbing then, please, think about this chapter as being about parkour and the next chapter awaits. However, if you have found yourself wondering 'Why *do* we do that?' but never dared to ask, think about standing on a ledge, think about surveying the terrain for your next jump and ask the question. What harm can be done by asking a question?

Of course, immense harm can be done because asking one question leads to asking another and another, and, before you know where you are, you are fomenting revolution. Not a destructive revolution, but creating constructive new approaches to empowering patients, introducing supportive structures and ultimately creating a healthier National Health Service. Whether you are a student, recently qualified health or social care practitioner or an experienced practitioner, you are being encouraged to show courage. The 6Cs, by the Commissioning Board Chief Nursing Officer and Department of Health Chief Nursing Adviser (2012), include Compassion, Communication, Commitment, Care, Competence and Courage. Courage is defined thus:

> Courage enables us to do the right thing for people we care for, to speak up when we have concerns and to have the personal strength and vision to innovate and to embrace new ways of working.' (Ibid.: 13)

The 'vision to innovate' requires us to see our work differently, to see it as it could be. The parkour practitioner who tries a new move or jump is aware that there is risk and the possibility of failure, but, without making the attempt, the purpose of doing parkour is rendered irrelevant. Similarly, in health and social care, if we are not prepared to be courageous in how we work, then our role as a health and social care professional is redundant. The possibility of failure is ever present in everything we do. We must systematically assess risk, plan effectively and communicate a vision to those with whom we work. That is good leadership and all good leaders begin by asking, 'Why *do* we do that?':

> It is the responsibility of leaders, in management and clinical roles, to manage the tension between the effects of industrialisation, regulation and task-related stress, and the precarious work of caring kindly and effectively for patients ... This may mean occasionally having the courage to subordinate financial and performance pressures to the need to ensure the right conditions for care, but that is not inevitable. (Ballatt and Campling, 2014: 181)

Conclusion

At the beginning of this chapter, we wrote about 'looking over the parapet'. Let us return to this now. If one assumes that what is over the parapet is bad, unpleasant or dangerous, then one will not look over the parapet. The assumption that what is over the parapet is bad, unpleasant and dangerous is enough to justify not looking over the parapet and to put forward an argument that what is over the parapet is enough to prevent one from looking over the parapet, ever again. So, how does it look now?

We hope that this chapter has helped you to think about your role and how that role is seen differently by you and by others. All our perspectives are built upon assumptions about the world and how we are positioned within it. The idea being that if we can learn to challenge our assumptions, then we may be able to reposition ourselves in the world. We will leave the last words to some positive reflections on parkour and what should now be the obvious parallels and lessons to be learnt from the practice of parkour, as a way not just to cope but also to thrive as a nurse:

> The freedom to move that Parkour enables was, and still is, a fundamental part of its philosophy. It's also what makes Parkour inherently political. Moving across the city in ways that it wasn't designed for is a liberating experience.
>
> Parkour is very much a reaction to the increased restriction of movement in modern cities: it allows [Parkour Practitioners] to rediscover their cities in an entirely new way, while also traversing architectural restrictions such as walls, fences and stair wells. (Mould, 2017)

References

Ballatt, J. and Campling, P. (2014) *Intelligent Kindness*. London: Royal College of Psychiatrists.

Boardman, J. and Roberts, G. (2014) *Risk, Safety and Recovery*. London: Centre for Mental Health and Mental Health Network, NHS Confederation.

Brookfield, S. (1995) *Becoming a Critically Reflective Teacher*. San Franciso, CA: Jossey-Bass.

Brown, N. (2017) *The Art of Displacement: Parkour as a Challenge to Social Perceptions of Body and Space*. London: Parkour Generations. Available at: www.aughty.org/pdf/art_of_displacement.pdf (accessed December 2017).

Casement, P. (1985) *On Learning from the Patient*. London: Routledge.

Commissioning Board Chief Nursing Officer and Department of Health (DH) Chief Nursing Adviser (2012) *Compassion in Practice*. Leeds: DH.

Department of Health (DH) (2007) *Independence, Choice and Risk: A Guide to Best Practice in Supported Decision-Making*. London: DH.

Ford, R. (2017) *How to Start Parkour: A Beginner's Guide*. London: Parkour Generations. Available at: https://apexmovement.com/blog/how-to-start-parkour-a-beginners-guide/ (accessed December 2017).

Francis, R. (2013) *Report of the Mid Staffordshire NHS Foundation Trust Public Inquiry, (The Francis Report): Executive Summary*. London: The Stationery Office.

Frankl, V. (2006 [1946]) *Man's Search for Meaning*. Boston, MA: Beacon Press.

Kubler-Ross, E. (1969) *On Death and Dying*. New York: Macmillan.

Mezirow, J. and Associates (1990) *Fostering Critical Reflection in Adulthood: A Guide to Transformative and Emancipatory Learning*. San Francisco, CA: Jossey-Bass.

Morgan, S. (2010a) 'Positive risk-taking: A basis for good risk decision-making', *Health Care Risk Report*, March.

Morgan, S. (2010b) 'Managing good risk decisions in mental health and social care', *Health Care Risk Report*, March.

Mould, O. (2017) 'The urban politics of parkour: How traceurs use sport to rediscover the city', *The Conversation*. Available at: http://theconversation.com/the-urban-politics-of-parkour-how-traceurs-use-sport-to-rediscover-the-city-62807 (accessed December 2017).

NHS Commissioning Board (2015) *New Care Models: Empowering Patients and Communities – A Call to Action for a Directory of Support*. London: NHS.

Parkour UK (2017) *What is Parkour?* Available at: http://parkour.uk/what-we-do/what-is-parkour/ (accessed December 2017).

Sport England (2017) *Active Lives Adult Survey*. London: Sport England.

10

How your Past Influences your Present

The Unconscious at Work

Cathy Constable

Chapter aims

- Understand the impact of the unconscious on the individual in the healthcare setting.
- Explore the concepts of transference and countertransference that can affect us at work.
- Appreciate the impact of our family relationships on our present-day relationships with colleagues.
- Understand the role of supervision in helping us keep boundaries.
- Develop your 'internal supervisor' and increase your resilience when working with teams and with service users.

As you read the following scenarios, think about your own experiences as you come into work to begin a shift.

Scenario 10.1   Samuel

Samuel was 15 minutes late for the night shift on A&E. It was his fourth night on, it had been a hot day and he had not been able to sleep well that day. His two children were on school holidays and had been playing noisily in their small garden. The ongoing row with his wife about wanting to move to a bigger house showed no signs of resolution.

They couldn't afford to increase the mortgage on their wages and Samuel was too tired to do overtime. He was on duty with Sally, a charge nurse. There was something about her that made him feel uncomfortable but he couldn't put his finger on it – he often found her approach lacking in confidence. When on duty with Sally, he always felt that he had to be on guard as if he didn't quite trust her or her decision-making. He had no reason to feel like this as colleagues rated her competence highly. It was Friday night and so was bound to be relentlessly busy. There was news that a serious road traffic accident (RTA) involving two children was about to come in. Samuel felt a sense of fear in the pit of his stomach. He took a deep breath, 'Ok, let's get on with it.' ...

Scenario 10.2   Melanie

Melanie sat in handover with a growing sense of annoyance and irritation. She had been qualified for 18 months and had enjoyed working on the acute mental health unit. Of course, it was busy, but she enjoyed working with the patients on the ward and generally within the team. She had, however, noticed over the past couple of months that she wasn't looking forward to work as much as she used to. Maybe the honeymoon period of being newly qualified was over? She thought about why she was annoyed (after all, they had drummed into them the importance of reflection during training). She knew that she felt mostly annoyed towards her colleague, Tony, but was unsure why. Every time they spoke, it seemed that he would disagree with her. Melanie felt that he often belittled her in front of others and that she would be left furious but unable to say anything. To feel helpless and that she is not being listened to is a common feeling for Melanie. It couldn't all be to do with him? It must be something to do with her, too? Anyway, she should be listening to handover and can't think about this now. She thought that, maybe, she needed to book in some supervision to talk about things – she hadn't been to supervision for ages ...

Introduction

Although these scenarios are fictitious, many readers will identify with these situations. Before we even start at work, there are numerous demands for our thoughts, attention and emotions. As discussed in earlier chapters, working within healthcare demands much emotional labour on the part of the nurse.

Chapter 3, 'Nursing: A Profession with too Many Masters?', the 'third person in the room' explores how the political dimension affects us as we work under the shadow of management, the organisation and the wider political climate. On a more personal level, we work within teams and with service users: a cast of characters with whom to interact and negotiate. We also bring to work with us the unconscious influences of our family of origin, potentially the blueprints to how we manage relationships in our adult world. We are also in a healthcare setting that involves working with patients who are anxious and frightened. Having to contain these influences on us (whether conscious or unconscious) can add to our personal emotional labour. Conversely, reflecting on the way in which we manage relationships we have at work can help us to learn about how we relate to others and, therefore, how to overcome unhelpful patterns of behaviour through an increase in our resilience and ability to cope during challenging times.

Transference and countertransference within the work setting: 'What is really going on here?'

The concepts of transference and countertransference are widely explored in the world of the psychotherapist–patient relationship but less so in the nurse–patient relationship. Some knowledge of these ideas can help lead us to some understanding of where our more difficult feelings at work may come from.

This chapter is based on the premise that the notion of the unconscious exists within us both individually and collectively within the organisations in which we work. The concept of the unconscious accepts that some of our mental content is outside our perception and, therefore, not accessible to our conscious minds but governs much of our behaviour. Freud described the unconscious mind as containing feelings, memories and thoughts that are inaccessible to our conscious awareness but influence our judgements, feelings or behaviour. He argued that much of the contents of the unconscious comprise of painful feelings, such as anxiety and conflict, and are repressed as they are too threatening for us to deal with. Freud believed that these feelings made themselves known through our dreams and slips ('Freudian slips'), and could be brought to consciousness through psychoanalysis.

'Transference' can be described as the unconscious emotional responses, experiences and expectations that we may bring to an interpersonal situation or relationship. There may be something familiar about a situation, subtle similarities between a present and past relationship or person that unconsciously triggers us to behave 'as if' that situation or person were in the present. Transference is used as a tool in psychoanalytic psychotherapy in order to help the patient explore the origins of unhelpful patterns in past relationships. This phenomena is driven by our past experience in relationships, particularly with authority figures. Sometimes, it is obvious why we behave like we do. A particularly overbearing mother may leave us with a fearful expectation that all women will behave in this way. At other times, we may repeat unhelpful behaviours (i.e., inappropriate relationship choices) because, although destructive, this feels more familiar than change.

So, why might an understanding of transference in the role of the nurse be useful? Jones (2005) highlights that understanding transference helps structure safe professional relationships. While the use of transference can be useful in the therapeutic relationship if used properly, it can also distort our perception of reality of the relationship with a patient as we transfer or project past feelings onto our encounters with that particular person. These feelings are not realistic or appropriate to the situation and can influence how we react or behave. An example of this may be the feelings that Melanie has towards Tony. She knows that she is overreacting but hasn't worked out why yet. You may be able to recall times when you (in hindsight) reacted inappropriately to a situation and then realised that you were influenced by patterns of unhelpful behaviour from your past that are often repeated in the present. Alternatively, your overreaction may have been pointed out by others, causing you to reflect on your behaviour. Jones points out that transference can be considered as a 'form of resistance or a mental defence to protect us from unresolved childhood conflicts' (2004: 14).

While transference describes past feelings projected on to another, countert-ransference is the term used to describe the unconscious response from those projec-tions, i.e. the unconscious response from the nurse to the patient or the response from Tony to Melanie's obvious irritation with him. Exploration of countertransference feelings can give us useful clues as to what is going on unconsciously in our patients and can help us work out 'whose feelings belong to who' in a situation.

How do we know when we are experiencing transference and countertransference at work? O'Kelly (1998) suggests that we need to pay attention to the appropriateness of our reactions to others in situations or encounters. This is not easy. How do we judge? Jones (2005) offers a useful checklist, as listed below.

Indications of Positive and Negative Transference and Countertransference in Nursing Relationships

- Strong feelings of affection or disaffection.

- Difficulties in setting limits or fixing rigid boundaries.

- A desire to please or avoid.

- Feeling either special or insignificant.

- Over- or under-involvement with a person.

- Feelings of marked comfort or discomfort with another.

- Preoccupation with another and/or power struggles.

Source: Jones (2005: 1183)

Reproduced with permission of John Wiley and Sons.

Unconscious defences created in the healthcare setting

As well as having difficult relationships with work colleagues, we also have to cope with working with patients who find themselves in challenging situations. As nurses, we work with patients who are in physical and emotional pain. Often both. Feelings such as anxiety, frustration and anger are ever present in the emotional maelstrom of the work environment. The nurse's role is to empathise with the patient and relate to their suffering in order to help contain it. Inevitably, we use our own experiences of suffering to be able to do this. We aim to respond to the patient with understanding and compassion. Ballatt and Campling (2011) describes the NHS as a relational system built on kinship. Being compassionate calls for intelligent kindness and the compassionate holding of the patient (or other) in our minds. In order to try and understand what another person is feeling, we need to put ourselves in their shoes, imagine what their experience might be like. It means that nurses have to make themselves vulnerable to the unknown experiences of others and, when patients are suffering, this can feel threatening, personally leaving us feeling anxious. This can lead to compassion fatigue and an attempt to protect ourselves by disengaging with patients in an attempt to distance ourselves from feelings of irritability and anger about the demands being made on us and feelings of hopelessness about our ability to cope.

Working with patients with physical problems also brings many anxieties to the surface for nursing staff. An understanding of transference and countertransference can also be useful in this setting and Menzies' (1959) influential research explored the unconscious emotional impact that nursing may have on us and how we may try to protect ourselves against anxiety.

Isabel Menzies, a psychoanalyst at the Tavistock Institute in London, was asked to investigate why there was a high degree of attrition in student nurses in a large London general hospital. As a consequence of her interviews with staff and observations, she describes the difficulties of working in healthcare at an unconscious level and how great emotional demands were placed on the nurses that could potentially overwhelm them with anxiety. Menzies drew on Kleinian psychoanalytic theory and suggested that working in close proximity to patients who may be suffering and dying, dealing with messy bodily functions, dealing with patients who had ambivalent feelings towards them (as they were both grateful and hostile because they were dependent on the nurse) aroused unconscious primitive desires and fears in the nurse.

This led to staff developing a personal and social defence system as a way of protecting themselves from the anxiety that nursing ill patients caused them. Staff either colluded with this system or left as their anxieties were too great, hence the high attrition rate. For example, Menzies observed that staff would collude in trying to distance themselves emotionally from patients by splitting the nurse–patient relationship by breaking down tasks into a list (I'll do all the blood pressures, you do the temperatures), therefore restricting contact with patients. She also described how patients were depersonalised by staff talking about patients by disease and not by name. Nurses were encouraged to stay emotionally detached and movement around the hospital at little notice was common. The management system was authoritarian but the managers were unable to create clear lines of authority or decision-making. It was often difficult to find out who was responsible for what. Although the paper is now several decades old, it is still very relevant and I urge you to read it and see if you recognise any of these organisational defence mechanisms happening now either in yourself or in the workplace. In a more recent exploration of Menzies's ideas, Armstrong and Rustin (2014) argue that, although the health system has changed considerably since the 1950s, the defensive practices still remain, with the aim of keeping the emotional experiences of the nursing task at a distance.

We only have to read the Francis Report (2013) in order to see history repeating itself in Menzies' criticism of the failure of the NHS as an organisation to help staff contain their anxieties. Francis criticises the fragmentation of the system, over-surveillance with target-setting and difficulties in being able to offer patient-centred care through often poor resourcing of clinical areas.

So, Menzies may offer us an explanation as to why working in health is stressful and what unconscious mechanisms may be involved to help us defend against the anxiety that work causes us. This general overview may resonate with you. Of course, it is also important to explore how we personally behave and react to others at work so as to gain some insight into our own patterns of behaviour. A useful way to explore this is in thinking about the workplace as an interpersonal or relational system. After all, as John Donne (1572–1631) wrote, 'No man is an island.'

Working in an interpersonal system

Those who have experience of working with families will be familiar with the notion of Family Systems Theory. Each family has unique complex family dynamics. This theory considers the family as an emotional unit and explores how family members communicate and relate to one another and what roles family members take on and are also coerced to take on by other family members. You may recognise some patterns in your behaviour during interactions with your family. Do you find yourself as the mediator or rescuer during family arguments? This behaviour can result due to a fear of family breakdown. Family members can often be polarised and so can be seen as 'good' or 'bad' members of the family. This is commonly known as 'scapegoating' and often the same family member is blamed for all the bad things that happen. In our example, Samuel finds Sally's approach lacking in confidence at times. Samuel's mother was an extremely shy person, with poor self-esteem. In contrast, his father had an over-dominant personality and could, at times, show his frustration about his wife's timid personality. This led Samuel to feel that he could not trust his mother to 'look out for him' or make good decisions about his life that he could trust, and working with Sally brought up these childhood feelings.

Many factors influence the role that we take on, such as past history of family dynamics and expectations in previous generations (i.e., all the women go into caring roles), how many siblings you have, the quality of the parental relationship and cultural influences, amongst others. Often, these roles are created unconsciously in order to create a balance in the family, and family members collude with the roles. As adults, these dynamics are often played out at family gatherings, where we can feel ourselves being pulled into the roles that we occupied when we were younger. This, of course, can be a positive or negative experience, depending on the roles you took (or were given) as a child. Bowen's influential model of family systems theory proposes that families are living organisms, with identifiable patterns of behaviour that are repeated, predictable and may undermine relationships within the family (Bowen, 1990). Members of the family are pulled between feeling part of the group and following these patterns and feeling separate from the family group. This tension, of course, is keenly felt during adolescence as we start to explore the wider world and try and separate from our families.

We may feel that we repeat these roles that we identify with at work. As organisations consist of groups of people, applying family systems theory to the workplace can be a useful way of understanding the relationships that we have between ourselves, as workers, at both a conscious or unconscious level. We are all part of a system, whether at home or at work, and, inevitably, these systems can overlap at times.

Senge (1999) advocates the importance of applying family systems theory when exploring relationship dynamics at work as a way of learning about ourselves and the roles that we transfer to work. This can help us understand and, therefore change, how we relate to others. Senge discusses the discipline of mental models describing this as 'turning the mirror inward' and learning to unearth our internal pictures of the world, to bring them to the surface and hold them up to scrutiny: Is what we think/believe really true? This also includes the ability to carry on 'learningful' conversations that balance inquiry and advocacy, where people expose their own thinking effectively and make that thinking open to the influence of others (ibid.: 9).

Although Senge writes for a general audience, his ideas are highly transferable to healthcare organisations. His concept of mental models, in particular, are of interest when thinking about relationships with colleagues and service users at work (1990). Exploring the mental models discipline asks us to reflect on our attitudes and assumptions that influence how we interact with each other. This involves us exploring our internal world and identifying maladaptive patterns of behaviour that we may fall into at work. On the flip side, we can also explore our strengths and engage in behaviour that is productive and helps us feel more in control and, therefore, increase our resilience at work.

So, how can we untangle our feelings and figure out what feelings belong to us and what feelings reside in those around us? How do we identify these patterns that can cause us anxiety and unhappiness at work? The negative patterns of behaviour that we fall into as a result of past difficult relationships are often unhelpful for us in the present day. Kerr and Minno (in Senge, 1999) suggest taking some time to ask yourself some questions about your relationship to your family of origin so as to try and explore the roots of this behaviour. If we look back at one of our examples, Melanie is concerned about her work relationship with Tony. She is feeling belittled by him but unable to say anything. Is this a pattern in her life? Melanie has acknowledged that she often feels like this with characters like Tony, whom she finds overbearing and overly critical. She has spoken to her colleagues about it but they tend to say that he is just trying to be helpful in his guidance.

Many of us can identify with this situation and it is difficult, if not impossible, to reflect on why we feel like we do in the heat of the moment. Emotions such as anger and frustration cloud our ability to think rationally. If you find yourself in similar situations, it may be useful to find some time to take part in Activity 10.1. Asking yourself the questions in the activity may help to identify patterns of behaviour that originate in your family of origin that you may want to address.

. . . .

Activity 10.1   Reflective Exercise on Family Origins

1. Who, at work, strongly reminds you of someone in your family of origin (including the extended family system)? What physical or behavioural attributes trigger you (i.e., facial expressions or features, gestures, particular behavioural habits, voice tones, etc.)?

2. How do you typically react (inwardly and externally) to that individual? How is this pattern of reacting similar to, or different from, your pattern of relating with the family of origin member?

3. Is the role that you are playing at work similar to, or different from, your family of origin role? You may not be replicating your family of origin role but you may be reacting against it.

4. Notice your behaviour in conflicts at work. When two people disagree, what is your response? Do you want to flee? Do you join in? Do you take the side of the one whom you perceive as weaker? Do you distance yourself from the fray? Do you mediate? Do you feel sick? Do you become quiet? Identify two or three aspects of your family history that seem relevant. Don't jump to any conclusions about these dynamics. You are still gathering information.

Source: Kerr and Minno in Senge (1999:217–2)

. . . .

Following on from this exercise Kerr and Minno suggest that those that undertake this exercise, if possible, write a short autobiography and genogram or family tree to gain a better understanding of their family of origins 'story'. This could relate back to relationships with siblings, parents and grandparents. Information could include that shown in Activity 10.2.

. . . .

Activity 10.2   Constructing a Family Tree

- Descriptions of your relationships with family members – what are the communication patterns?
- The roles that you and others played in the family.
- What are the families' significant events/experiences – major illness, loss?
- What are the important family values and beliefs?
- Are there any spoken or unspoken family rules?

. . . .

Exploring these issues may give rise to the identification of the origin of certain behaviours or the identification of long-held beliefs that are no longer relevant to you and, in fact, hampering your personal development.

Kerr and Minno also suggest that, if possible, you should speak to members of your family. Tell them that you are doing your family tree or autobiography. If this is possible, you may be able to explore the questions above: How did your parents get on with their parents? What were their attitudes and beliefs about the world and how to interact with it? What are the family scripts and rules that have been passed down the generations – are they helpful to you now? This exercise comes with a health warning. Of course, this is an extremely sensitive exercise to embark on and needs to be undertaken with a spirit of curiosity, in a non-judgemental, non-blaming environment. Kerr and Minno (in Senge, 1999: 272) point out the golden rule of family-of-origin work: 'Its purpose is to change you and not others.'

Undertaking this exercise may help you understand better the unconscious motivation for your behaviour with certain people or in certain situations. Then you can try new approaches and see what works for you so as to ensure a more positive outcome. The key then is to try and change how you react.

Melanie took some time to think about her work relationship with Tony and whether it brought up any patterns from the past. She spoke to an old school friend who knew her well when she was growing up. Melanie has a sister, Jane, who is five years older. As children, Melanie always felt that she was 'second best' to her sister. Jane was very academic and excelled at school, going on to become a lawyer, like their father. Their parents were obviously proud of Jane, calling her the 'academic one', whilst Melanie was the 'practical one'. Melanie struggled academically and felt that she always lived in Jane's shadow at school. She would not describe their relationship as close then or now. Jane also suffered poor health as a child experiencing asthma that necessitated frequent hospital visits. Melanie would describe Jane as bossy and felt that she left little room for her own point of view in their frequent arguments. Melanie felt that their mother would always defend Jane, asking Melanie to stop arguing for fear of bringing on an asthma attack. Melanie noted that when she spoke to Tony and she again felt those old feelings of not being listened to and that there was no point in putting her views across.

However, there is no denying that changing years of ingrained patterns is difficult and it is easy to be pulled back into old patterns of behaviour at times of stress. Practising mindfulness can give the opportunity to be more proactive in a situation than just being reactive. Finding that space between thought and reacting can give us the opportunity to change our behaviour. In Covey's foreword to Pattakos & Dundon's (2017) book *Prisoner of our Thoughts*, he refers to a quotation (p. vi), attributed to Frankl when telling of how he survived the holocaust by developing a personal sense of meaning and purpose:

> Between stimulus and response there is a space. In that space is our power to choose our response. In our response lies our growth and our freedom.

Using writing as a tool to reflect

Chapter 6 introduced Johns' (1995) 'Model of Structured Reflection' and the idea of creating space for reflection. In his latest book about becoming a reflective practitioner, Johns explores ways of 'bringing the mind home' through writing:

> To write I find a quiet eddy out of the fast current of life, to pause, to muse, to clear and let go of the mind and open the body to recall the experience, to create a space where I can get back into the experience with all my senses. Yet in the busy and material world in which we live this may not be easy. Our minds are often full of stuff that distracts us. Like a juggler trying to keep eight plates spinning. Generally people do not take time to slow down and press the pause button. Having the mind full of stuff also offers an excuse not to look at the self in any deep way. (2017: 21)

Johns (2017) writes eloquently and in depth about the usefulness of the process of writing. He advocates the use of writing or journaling about our experiences as a medium to reflect on. The process of writing encourages the organisations of thoughts, can help work through feelings and therefore can be cathartic. If we write about painful experiences or need to be self-critical then this can be more challenging but valuable. You may like to use the exercise in Activity 10.3 in order to try and work through a difficult situation at work or with a colleague or patient.

....

Activity 10.3   Writing Exercise

Think about a work situation that you may want to write about. Make sure that you will be undisturbed for 20 minutes or so. Get a pen and some paper or use a PC, whichever you prefer, and find a comfortable seated position. Take a few minutes to relax yourself and bring your mind home. To do this, you could practise some mindfulness techniques or engage in some deep breathing for a couple of minutes. Don't worry about having to clear your mind. If a thought pops up, just acknowledge it but don't engage with it. You could close your eyes and focus on the breath – count it in and out slowly. When you feel ready, write about your experience, describe what happened in detail, your surroundings, what you did, other's reactions. How did you feel? What emotions surfaced? What memories did the situation bring up? Don't worry too much about making sense or grammar. There is no right or wrong in this exercise. You are not writing an assignment! This is just for you. Stop when you are ready.

   If this process feels too threatening, you could write about yourself in the third person or as a character. You may like to have a short break and then reflect on what you have written. How does it feel reading what you have written? Are there any new insights into your behaviour or that of others? What was useful about the exercise for you? Are there any patterns emerging in your behaviour? What might the origin of these be? Can you identify which feelings are yours and which feelings you have taken on from others?

....

The Value and Therapeutic Benefit of Writing

- Paints a rich descriptive canvas for reflection.

- Focuses attention on one's practice and recognising significance within the unfolding situation.

- Develops perception.

- Enables self to become aware of self and others within the context of the practice environment/connection with self and with others (empathy).

- Is cathartic/healing/transformative.

- Points to problems and contradictions with values.

- Others can relate to because of its subjective and contextual nature.

Source: Johns (2017:31)

Building supportive clinical supervision

As well as working with colleagues who challenge us, we also work with patients and situations that challenge us and have an impact on our emotions as they strike a chord with us in some way or another. In our example, Samuel dreads the day his children might be involved in an accident. Working in a stressful and busy accident and emergency department can make it appear as if there is a disproportionate number of accidents. Part of feeling stressed is a difficulty in keeping perspective.

It is worth repeating that, as nurses, we bring our emotional selves to our work with patients. An understanding of what are our emotions and what belongs to the patient can be useful in maintaining our professional boundaries and containing our anxieties. The relationships we have with patients are unique and can bring us much role satisfaction. However, there are times when we struggle. Our role is to build relationships, often with people who don't want to engage with us. As nurses, we still continue to engage when we are dismissed and rejected by what we may perceive as unappreciative patients. This can take a toll on us emotionally. During these times, it is easy just to carry on keeping our heads down in the busy day job. Although it can feel like an extra burden to talk about these issues, it could be argued that this is the very time that we need to do so.

The concept of clinical supervision is embedded in mental health nursing but less so in adult nursing. The NMC highlight the importance of the process of reflection on our practice in order to ensure that we maintain a high standard of care, and it encourages us to practise effectively: 'reflect and act on any feedback you receive to improve your practice' (NMC, 2015: 7). Esterhuizan and Freshwater describe clinical supervision and reflective practice as interdependent and clinical supervision as 'a flexible and dynamic structure in which to continuously deconstruct and reconstruct clinical practice' (2008: 120).

Clinical Supervision

The Royal College of Nursing (n.d.) describes 'clinical supervision' as:

> an activity that brings skilled supervisors and practitioners together in order to reflect upon their practice. It is a time for you, as a nurse or midwife, to think about your knowledge and skills and how they may be developed to improve care. It has been described as providing education for the nurse and protection for the client. (p.1)

Effective clinical supervision that balances challenge and support needs an ethical structure so that supervisees feel safe in the relationship to reflect on issues. It is important that you choose a supervisor whom you feel that you can trust and be open with. It is also important to set the 'ground rules' when you first meet. The structure for supervision comes from agreed contracts that set clear boundaries and outline goals, roles and responsibilities (Ferguson, 2005). It may be that your Trust has a clinical supervision policy or guidelines. The careful development of a trusting relationship is key to the success of clinical supervision.

In order to be productive, supervision needs to have a safe space where the supervisee can be held and supported. This space may also become uncomfortable at times when we are challenged, disagreements may occur and anxiety provoked when resolutions to situations are not yet known. All of this can only be tolerated if the supervision space has the capacity to contain these experiences (Page and Woskett, 1994).

Hawkins and Shohet (2006) advocate experiencing good quality supervision at the beginning of nursing careers and it therefore becoming an integral part of the lifelong learning process. Regular use of supervision can encourage the development of an 'internal supervisor', allowing more autonomous working with increased confidence in decision-making abilities as more experience is gained in the healthcare setting (Casement, 1990: 9). The idea of the internal supervisor is that you can take the lessons you learn about yourself from clinical supervision and apply them in practice, as you are working. However, there is a risk that, without careful handling, supervision may cross over the boundary to therapy.

Yegdich (1999) questioned how supervision can be differentiated from therapy because, although they have different aims, they share a similar goal of personal and professional growth. He argued that this differentiation is important for supervision to be a credible process in nursing and stresses the importance of the supervisor focusing on the tripartite relationship between the supervisor, supervisee and patient. Hawkins and Shohet agree and describe the supervisory relationship as 'a container that holds the helping relationship within the therapeutic triad' (2006: 3). Of course, the supervisor needs to be sensitive to the supervisee's needs and may need to discuss the issue of further support, if appropriate. If you or your supervisor do feel that boundaries have been crossed and you have started to use supervision as therapy, then it may be time to seek out some counselling for yourself.

Conclusion

This chapter has explored the importance of getting to know ourselves through the process of reflecting on our family of origin and the stories and patterns of behaviour contained there. Bringing our unconscious thoughts, feelings and behaviours to consciousness through the process of reflection can help give us a better understanding of why we behave like we do with colleagues and service users in the workplace. Good clinical supervision can help give us the space to reflect on our roles. A chance to step back and explore the motivations for our behaviour in the safe space of clinical supervision can help us internalise the reflective nature of supervision.

This, is turn, can lead to greater feelings of resilience in the workplace as we are able to reflect in the moment during the workday, or 'in action' as Schön (1983) described it. A greater sense of ourselves can lead us to feel that we are more in control of our situation, leading to decreased feelings of stress and greater role satisfaction.

References

Armstrong, D. and Rustin, M. (2014) *Social Defences against Anxiety*. London: Karnac Books.

Ballatt, J. and Campling, P. (2011) *Intelligent Kindness: Reforming the Culture of Healthcare*. London: Royal College of Psychiatrists.

Bowen, M. (1990) *Family Therapy in Clinical Practice*. New York: Jason Aronson.

Casement, P. (1990) *Further Learning from the Patient: The Analytic Space and Process*. London: Tavistock/Routledge.

Esterhuizan, P. and Freshwater, D. (2008) 'Clinical supervision and reflective practice', in D. Freshwater, B.J. Taylor and G. Sherwood (eds), *International Textbook of Reflective Practice in Nursing*. Chichester: Blackwell.

Ferguson, K. (2005) 'Professional supervision'. In D. Best and M. Rose (eds) *Transforming Practice through Clinical Education, Professional Supervision and Mentoring, Churchill Livingstone*, pp. 293–308. Edinburgh Elsevier.

Francis, R. (2013) *Report of the Mid Staffordshire NHS Foundation Trust Public Inquiry*. London: The Stationery Office.

Hawkins, P. and Shohet, R. (2006) *Supervision in the Helping Professions*. Maidenhead: Open University Press.

Johns, C. (1995) 'Framing learning through reflection within Carper's fundamental ways of knowing in nursing', *Journal of Advanced Nursing*, 22 (2): 226–34.

Johns, C. (2017) *Becoming a Reflective Practitioner*. Hoboken, NJ: Wiley-Blackwell.

Jones, A. (2004) 'Transference and countertransference', *Perspectives in Psychiatric Care*, 40: 13–19.

Jones, A. (2005) 'Transference, counter-transference and repetition: Some implications for nursing practice', *Journal of Clinical Nursing*, *14*: 1177–84.

Menzies Lyth, I.E.P. (1959) 'The functions of social systems as a defence against anxiety: A report on a study of the nursing service of a general hospital', *Human Relations*, *13*: 95–121. Reprinted in I.E.P. Menzies Lyth, *Containing Anxiety in Institutions: Selected Essays*, Vol. 1. London: Free Association Books, 1988.

Nursing & Midwifery Council (NMC) (2015) *The Code: Professional Standards of Practice and Behaviour for Nurses and Midwives*. London: NMC.

O'Kelly, G. (1998) 'Counter-transference in the nurse patient relationship: A review of the literature', *Journal of Advanced Nursing*, *28*: 391–7.

Page, S. and Wosket, V. (1994) *Supervising the Counsellor. A Cyclical Model*. London: Routledge.

Pattakos, A. and Dundon, E. (2017) *Prisoners of our Thoughts*, 3rd edition. New York: McGraw-Hill Education.

Royal College of Nursing (RCN) (n.d.) *Clinical Supervision I*. Available at: https://www.rcn.org.uk/get-help/rcn-advice/clinical-supervision (accessed 12 March 2018).

Schön, D.A. (1983) *The Reflective Practitioner*. London: Temple Smith.

Senge, P.M. (1990) *The Fifth Discipline. The Art and Practice of the Learning Organization*. London: Random House.

Senge, P.M. (1999) *The Dance of Change: The Challenges of Sustaining Momentum in Learning Organizations*. New York: Currency/Doubleday.

Yegdich, T. (1999) 'Lost in the crucible of supportive clinical supervision: Supervision is not therapy', *Journal of Advanced Nursing*, *29* (5): 1265–75.

11

Conclusion

Going Green – A Toolkit to Support Sustainable Practice

Peter J. Martin

Conclusion aims

- Revisit the contemporary context of health and social care.
- Consider the consequences of failing to respond positively within this environment.
- Look at what is meant by 'sustainability'.
- Begin to place some ideas into a 'toolbox' for future use.

The service user as the voice of reason

The focus of health and social care should always be the person who seeks our assistance. We can call that person a patient, a service user, a client but, whatever title we use, they remain the person who is seeking our help.

As people who work in health and social care, we live daily with the orderly chaos of many of our busy hospitals. The beeping machines, the electronic documentation the paraphernalia of the nurse or the doctor are all commonplace. To the person entering our services, this is a very different and strange environment: a forbidding environment. In order for the person to get through this experience, they need a friendly face and an approachable demeanour: a metaphorical hand to hold.

If we cannot cope and thrive in a health and social care service that is for us to address, it is neither the fault nor the responsibility of the person in front of us. The person with cardiac arrhythmia or experiencing voice-hearing for the first time should not feel the brunt of our daily battles with 'the management' or 'staffing levels'. This is our emotional labour.

It seems appropriate, therefore, to start the Conclusion by listening to the person who is the end user of our services. In Case Study 11.1, a colleague and service user with whom we work offers us an insight into what he wants from health and social care services. This is a calm and thoughtful voice of reason that expresses reasonable expectation. Whilst we need to consider every point that is made, I have highlighted the last three, in particular, which are very pertinent to this book.

Case Study 11.1   The Needs of the Service User

What I want nurses to know or understand in order to give me the best care to aid my recovery:

- A basic understanding of a person's history, where this is relevant to improving care.

- Demonstrable personal qualities that include a natural disposition towards compassion.

- A sense of humour when and where appropriate, and a cheerful disposition.

- An understanding of local and international events, factors and developments and the ability to see how these can be utilised in order to improve patient care.

- An ability to champion patient needs during times of adversity or incapacity.

- Recognition of recovery as being different for each person, alongside the ability to adapt your practice to the needs of the recovering person.

- An ability to converse and communicate effectively with decision–makers in other areas of health and social care for the benefit of patients.

- Knowing that a person's recovery is not an open-and-shut case and is for their whole life, and realising that each person's recovery is an individual journey, and being able to provide as much individualised care as possible for each recovering patient.

- An ability to recognise, neutralise and circumvent negative structures and elements within cultures, institutions and societies that are damaging to patient care, compassion and recovery.

- A willingness to support your colleagues and patients at all times by leaving irrelevant, toxic and unhelpful attitudes, beliefs and actions outside of work.

- Understanding your [nurse's] importance as frontline healthcare professionals and being able to resist and thwart pressure from those above you in the hierarchy.

Source: Robert, Service User

This conclusion brings together content from the preceding chapters in order to offer a coherent proposition for positive change. The chapter offers the opportunity to revisit and integrate different techniques and strategies in ways that suit the individual practitioner.

More specifically, the chapter looks at the nature of sustainable change – that is, change that can be maintained without further depletion of limited energy resources. What we want to propose is that any changes must be simple enough to be easily adopted within everyday working practices. Changes should not require physical infrastructures or specific training and development in order to be of benefit.

We should be clear, we are not indicating that training and development is not useful or relevant; that is, after all, our core purpose as nurse educators. What we are advocating is that the techniques included in this book are available to all with the most minimal of input. By all means take these ideas forward, study them and learn more about them but, in the first instance, try them out and see if they are useful in meeting your individual needs at this time.

Health and social care in the UK

The focus of the preceding chapters has been on finding ways by which practitioners can more effectively manage in the current health and social care climate. This climate has been explored and explained in some form in all the chapters. So, bringing these arguments together, we can characterise this climate in the ways shown in Figure 11.1.

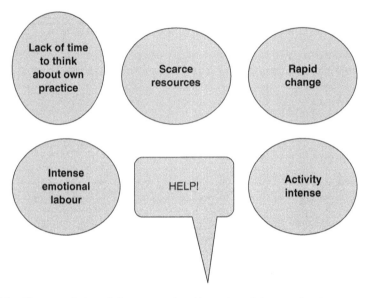

Figure 11.1   Characteristics of the current health and social care climate

Scarce resources

Politicians will continue to dispute the actual spend on the NHS. This is nothing new and will continue, at least, for as long as the NHS is publicly funded. However, the experience of staff at the patient interface is that they feel that they have not got adequate human or physical resources. This is experienced through the inability to discharge effectively the job for which they are employed in a manner that meets their professional code of practice and from which they may derive satisfaction.

Rapid change

it became clear that future shock is no longer a distantly potential danger, but a real sickness from which increasingly large numbers already suffer. This psycho-biological condition can be described in medical and psychiatric terms. It is the disease of change. (Toffler, 1970: 10)

In order to demonstrate the prior knowledge that we should have about the impact of change, this quote from Toffler was written nearly half a century ago. Toffler recognised that the pace of change would have a bewildering and disorientating impact on individuals and that adaptation was critical to survival.

The pace of change in health and social care is no different to any other part of society and health and social care practitioner must learn to work within a dynamic environment. Changes may be occurring internally with new technologies and organisational structures or externally with the changing health and social care needs of the population. Wherever the source of the change, practitioners must adapt their practices on a continuing basis:

Change is not merely necessary to life – it is life. (Toffler, 1970: 176)

Activity intense

Practitioners working in health and social care services need to be able to manage periods of intense activity, although, arguably, in contemporary services, periods of lesser intensity are more likely to be the exception.

In order to manage in busy services, we *think on our feet* so that we can deal with rapidly changing situations. Schön (1983) contended that this *thinking on our feet* was a highly logical and systematic process that the ability to *reflect-in-action* was inadequately valued by a society driven by a desire for technical rationality. Schön (1987) wrote about the importance of the professional's ability to respond rapidly to events. He described the 'zones of indeterminacy', which were to be found in practice and for which conventional ways of thinking and behaving were inadequate. The absence of formulaic problem-solving in such environments requires practitioners to develop creative and innovative ways to resolve problems.

Such creative problem-solving skills, Schön contended, were the bedrock of professional practice. But, in order to effectively 'reflect in action', we need to be able to learn from our own experiences by taking time regularly to think about our practice.

Lack of time to think about your own practice

> Time, and the attention and communication it allows, is increasingly unavailable in a modern NHS characterised by the drive to speed up treatment processes and to save money by providing the minimum numbers of staff. Time and human resources pressures frequently conspire to direct attention to procedures, to fragmented targets and tasks, and away from genuine engagement with patients. (Ballatt and Campling, 2011: 111)

An inevitable consequence of the high level of activity commonplace in health and social care services is the absence of time to stop and think about our practice. Without this time, we cease to be able to learn from our experiences.

It is an often cited aphorism that one can have 20 years of experience or one year of experience 20 times. At the point where we cease to have the time or energy to pause and think about our practice is when we move towards the latter condition. If we are not learning from our experiences, we risk repeating the same mistakes over and over again. By simply repeating experiences without any time to reflect, we stop growing as people and the job we aspired to do becomes a routine, like threading washers on a rod.

It is important to emphasise that this is not intended to belittle highly skilled and knowledgeable practitioners from all health and social care professions. The purpose of this argument is to highlight the significance of learning from practice in the development of professional knowledge; and the building of a repertoire of knowledge and skills that can be utilised on the messy problems of everyday practice that don't accord with standardised procedures and policies (Schön, 1983, 1987).

A practical example, with which all nurses will be familiar, is pre-registration nurse education. The NMC (2010) state that, 'R5.2.3 – AEIs must ensure there are at least 2300 hours of practice learning', which is 50 per cent of the programme of study. Consider if every hour of the 2300 hours was simply repeated without any further learning taking place. You may feel that this is a completely absurd statement, but we need to consider why this is any different for the qualified practitioner who must also continue to learn from their practice.

Intense emotional labour

All of the above now have to be considered within the context of a human service. Health and social care has always had a high level of emotional labour (Hochschild, 1983): this is unchanged.

Of the five points identified in Figure 11.1, this is arguably the most static in terms of input. Patients have always exhibited stress and distress and nurses have always responded in a compassionate manner. The presentation of, for example, a fractured femur is generally similar over time.

What may have changed is the level of activity and acuity. Health and social care workers are dealing with a greater throughput of people in need and the demands on them to manage emotional labour effectively are consequently increased. Such an increase has not been born alongside a concomitant increase in effective support and supervision networks.

Returning to the last three of Robert's (service user) 'reasonable requests' of health and social care staff:

- An ability to recognise, neutralise and circumvent negative structures and elements within cultures, institutions and societies that are damaging to patient care, compassion and recovery.
- A willingness to support your colleagues and patients at all times by leaving irrelevant, toxic and unhelpful attitudes, beliefs and actions outside of work.
- Understanding your [nurse's] importance as frontline healthcare professionals and being able to resist and thwart pressure from those above you in the hierarchy.

These three points demand that, if we are to be a positive force in our engagement with patients, we must work within the five points listed in Figure 11.1 and find a more sustainable way of coping and thriving.

Based on scenarios and the voices of practitioners throughout this book, we have offered an assumption that many health and social care practitioners are struggling to get through their day. For many who do get through their day, the end of the day is often one of physical and mental exhaustion.

Reacting to circumstances

The current environment within the health and social care sector would seem to present practitioners with significant challenges. In order to survive this environment, practitioners have to determine a way forward for themselves. There would appear to be four alternative strategies that practitioners can adopt:

1. Leave

Many nurses and midwives chose to leave nursing and take on different roles that they find are less stressful;

> The change in the overall number of nurses and midwives registered with us is largely driven by an increase in the number of people leaving the register. (NMC, 2017: 8)

In Chapter 4, Cathy Constable looked at some of the things that inspired us to become nurses. There are, I am sure, many nurses who have left the profession and have found equal fulfilment in new careers. Nonetheless, there are many former nurses who are not able to find the same job satisfaction that they had when they were nursing.

2.   Do an inadequate or poor job

In the Introduction, I noted that one of the assumptions underpinning this book was that no nurse entered the profession with the intention of doing harm. There are presently significant systemic issues in the environment in which nurses work that create the conditions and cultures in which poor practice can emerge and flourish. There have been a number of recent reports, highlighting poor practices in health and social care. The Francis Report (2013) is one example where systemic failures are highlighted:

> The report has identified numerous warning signs which cumulatively, or in some cases singly, could and should have alerted the system to the problems developing at the Trust. That they did not has a number of causes, among them:
>
> * A culture focused on doing the system's business – not that of the patients;
> * An institutional culture which ascribed more weight to positive informa-tion about the service than to information capable of implying cause for concern;
> * Standards and methods of measuring compliance which did not focus on the effect of a service on patients;
> * Too great a degree of tolerance of poor standards and of risk to patients;
> * A failure of communication between the many agencies to share their knowl-edge of concerns;
> * Assumptions that monitoring, performance management or intervention was the responsibility of someone else;
> * A failure to tackle challenges to the building up of a positive culture, in nurs-ing in particular but also within the medical profession;
> * A failure to appreciate until recently the risk of disruptive loss of corporate memory and focus resulting from repeated, multi-level reorganisation. (Francis 2013: 4)

Nurses individually are accountable for, and should be accountable for, their own practice. They are also individually accountable for preventing bad practice directly or through whistle-blowing: to be silent is to be complicit. Taking account of the individual nurse's accountability, punishing this individual without addressing the systemic issues that created the climate in which bad practice flourished, is not con-structive and counterproductive.

3.   Sacrifice personal health

It seems a terrible irony that so many nurses become damaged whilst working in a health and social care service that demands compassion from its entire staff. Nonetheless, we work with staff who are being damaged by the health and social care system daily.

When we work with qualified staff undertaking continuous professional development programmes, we spend a great deal of time also working with the defences that staff have put in place to protect themselves. We see this through a cynical, demeaning and self-deprecating sense of humour, evidenced through phrases such as: 'The management, well that's a joke in itself ...' or 'Well, I'm only a nurse, so what do I know.'

It is this pessimistic attitude towards nursing that becomes the received wisdom of our students, the future nurses and managers of the health and social care service. For example, when teaching about negotiated care planning, students have asserted that negotiation did not take place where they worked previously; patients were expected to sign the completed care plan. The attitudes expressed by some nurses with whom we work have not arisen spontaneously. Rather, they are constructed on years of supressed emotions for which there has been inadequate organisational support or compassion.

4.   Undertake paradigmatic change

The first three options would seem to be regrettable, damaging, unhealthy or all three. So, is there an alternative?

The work of Brookfield was introduced in Chapter 3, where causal assumptions in relation to Jenny's scenario were discussed. Brookfield (1995) presented three types of assumptions:

- Causal assumptions relate to how things work and how they can be changed.
- Prescriptive assumptions explore what we think ought to be happening in a particular situation.
- Paradigmatic assumptions are the most deeply embedded assumptions that reflect our world view.

> Paradigmatic assumptions are the hardest of the three kinds [of assumptions] to uncover. They are the basic structuring axioms we use to order the world into fundamental categories. We may not recognize them as assumptions, even after they've been pointed out to us. Instead we insist that they're objectively valid renderings of reality, the facts as we know them to be true. (Ibid.: 2)

Brookfield argues that people operate through paradigmatic assumptions about the world. Consequently, if our assumption is that the system in which we work is all-powerful and that nothing we can do will change things, then we will act accordingly. This may be demonstrated by a practitioner adopting a role of passivity and unquestioning obedience to managers.

Whilst acknowledging that power is not vested equally, Brookfield urges us to challenge the assumptions that govern our behaviours. If we take the time to uncover the assumptions by which we act and ask critical questions about their legitimacy, then we can begin a paradigmatic shift that will allow us to be a practitioner who is, in Robert's words, *able to resist and thwart pressure from those above you in the hierarchy*.

Sustainability

With paradigmatic change comes a new way of looking at the workplace and how we engage with this environment. However, this, in itself, is inadequate to allow health and social care professionals to 'cope and thrive'. At the same time, it is important to begin to put things in place to promote positive and sustainable change in our behaviours as well as our thinking.

'Sustainable,' in general usage, is defined by the *Oxford English Dictionary* (2011) as:

- Able to be sustained …
- Conserving an ecological balance by avoiding depletion of natural resources.

'Sustainable change,' therefore, should not be about complex infrastructures or training. Such endeavours will use up energy and be swiftly dropped the minute that the service becomes busy.

For example, in order to work more efficiently in a busy service, you may feel that to be in possession of more effective time-management skills would be a useful asset. On the NHS.UK website, the following 'Easy Time Management Tips' (NHS, 2017) are recommended. These are all valuable, important and well-researched skills in time management and are commendable.

Easy Time-Management Tips

1. Work out goals
2. Make a list
3. Focus on results
4. Have a lunch break
5. Prioritise important tasks

6. Practice the 4 Ds:

    1. Delete

    2. Do

    3. Delegate

    4. Defer

However, a well-planned and goal-driven day can quickly get knocked off course following an unexpected admission, a difficult delayed discharge or an outbreak of diarrhoea and vomiting in a neighbouring ward. An inability to achieve a tidy goal-driven day on one occasion you can overlook, but if this becomes a recurring pattern then you are less and less likely to make further attempts. You may begin to think that attempting to improve your time-management skill is futile and that you will always be reacting to circumstances and firefighting.

Reproduced with permission.

Whatever changes we make to our practice, they must be sustainable. Moving from a generic to a more specific definition of 'sustainability' might help explain what needs to happen. 'Social sustainability' is defined as:

> The ability of a community to develop processes and structures which not only meet the needs of its current members but also support the ability of future generations to maintain a healthy community. (*Business Directory*, 2017)

Within this definition are embedded some helpful components that we can use to explore social sustainability within the terms of this book;

1. We can consider the *community* as a group sharing a common set of values and goals. For example, this may be the 'nursing community' or the 'ward' or simply a group of health and social care practitioners.
2. *Processes and structures* are those tools that have been discussed in the preceding chapters.
3. The aim of this book is to meet the *current needs* of practitioners in order for them to cope and thrive, but also …
4. Ensuring that *future generations* of our students learn how to cope and thrive from the skilled practitioners within their practice placements.
5. Finally, the importance of creating a *healthy community* of health and social care practitioners in order that they can deliver a high-quality service to patients for whom they are caring.

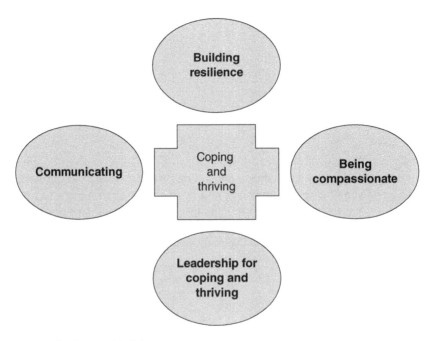

Figure 11.2 Coping and thriving

Some ideas for a toolkit to support sustainable practice

Building resilience

> Resilience is the process of effectively negotiating, adapting to, or managing significant sources of stress or trauma. Assets and resources within the individual, their life and environment facilitate this capacity for adaptation and 'bouncing back in the face of adversity. Across the life course, the experience of resilience will vary. (Windle, 2011: 163)

Using Windle's definition, 'resilience' is seen, not as a product or something to be attained, but as a process that is continually negotiated, adapted to or managed. This definition is consistent with the goals of this book. Throughout, we have offered a number of different strategies and tools on the assumption that such tools are always context-dependent. What works for some people will not work for others; what doesn't work today might work next week.

In Chapter 3, Martin and Harrison looked at Rotter's (1954) Locus of Control. It was postulated that, through thinking about the principles of the Locus of Control, we can begin to understand how we are engaging with the environment. Do we feel:

1. Powerless to the extent that we have no opportunity to improve our own circumstances or those of the people for whom we are caring? (Externalised locus of control)

2. Lacking in extensive power, but still able to influence our immediate environ-
    ment to provide better care and a more self-fulfilling environment? (Internalised
    locus of control)

Bringing to the surface our awareness of one's self within the environment is
essential to being able to develop a more internalised locus of control. At the start
of this chapter, Robert exhorted nurses about our own 'importance as frontline
healthcare professionals and being able to resist and thwart pressure from those
above you in the hierarchy'.

In Chapter 5, Caroline Barratt and Tess Wagstaffe explored mindfulness as a way
of becoming present amidst distraction and chaos, to recognise, as they describe it,
'moments in which we can perhaps reconnect with why we do what we do and, in
turn, find satisfaction and pleasure within our role as a nurse'.

Constable, in Chapter 4, introduces 'Intelligent Kindness' (Ballatt and Campling,
2011), which urges us to adopt an attitude that 'unsentimentally values kinship and
kindness, understanding their creative, motivating power' (ibid.: 175). Such an
attitude may help us explore more openly the impact of our emotional labour.

Whilst, as nurse lecturers, we are regularly told by nurses that they don't have the
time to reflect, Wood's considered overview of a number of reflective approaches in
Chapter 6 serves as a reminder that reflection is critical to learning from our own
experiences. Continuing learning in practice helps to build a portfolio of responses
to the unique, value-laden problems regularly faced within practice. A strong
personal portfolio enables us to manage the surprises that practice regularly presents.

Being compassionate

> Compassion is how care is given through relationships based on empathy,
> respect and dignity – it can also be described as intelligent kindness, and is
> central to how people perceive their care. (Commissioning Board Chief Nursing
> Officer and DH Chief Nursing Adviser, 2012: 13)

Barratt and Wagstaffe's outline of applied mindfulness in Chapter 5 can help to
develop a more compassionate approach to health and social care. When overwhelmed by the 'noise', the activity and the raw expressed emotion of practice areas,
to have the ability to be 'present' rather than just 'functioning', makes the person in
front of us a human being once again.

A precursor to being compassionate is to show some degree of self-compassion.
In Chapter 7, Tess Wagstaffe and Ness Woodstock-Dennis looked at self-
compassion and how mindfulness can be used to develop self-compassion. They
are very explicit that self-compassion is not being selfish or egocentric but is being
kind to oneself.

A significant innovation within health and social care services is the development
of Schwartz Rounds, which Mary Kennedy discussed in Chapter 1. Such an
approach brings people together in a spirit of compassion, not to problem-solve
but to better understand the lived experience of doing emotional labour. It is useful

to couple this idea with an understanding of the Wounded Healer, which Constable describes in Chapter 4.

Leadership for coping and thriving

> The NHS is facing a whole array of unprecedented changes and challenges. There are resource constraints, new demands, new institutions, and high expectations from patients and the public that service and care will be delivered efficiently, effectively and with compassion. To meet such an array of needs it is recognised that appropriate leadership is vital. (Storey and Holti, 2013: 4)

Leadership can be delivered through the organisation. Those leading and those managing are not necessarily the same people. In Chapter 2, Steve Wood offers three creative strategies for innovative leadership: creative change (Mueller, 2017), the 'struggle switch' (Harris, 2006) and 'change disrupters' (Carlson, 2017).

In Chapter 6, Wood argues for the importance of the marginal gains associated with Syed's (2016) 'black box' thinking. When considered alongside a strengthened internalised locus of control, marginal gains can make a real difference to how health and social care practitioners cope and thrive in stressed workplaces.

The fundamental attributes of parkour, described by Martin Harrison and Peter J. Martin in Chapter 9, offer a light-hearted way of viewing the seemingly intransigent problems of leading within health and social care. The next time you are in practice, you may want to think of yourself as balancing on a parapet, seemingly defying gravity but being able to see the world from a completely new perspective. In this chapter, Harrison and Martin also discuss how we make meaning out of the seemingly endless flow of information within health and social care.

As Kennedy describes in Chapter 8, leaders need to form mutually beneficial partnerships with other professionals and with patients and their families. The excerpt from the Francis Report cited earlier noted that there existed a 'culture focused on doing the system's business – not that of the patients' (Francis, 2013). As health and social care practitioners, we should be working in partnership with patients in order to diminish the 'them and us' culture prevalent in some areas of practice.

Communicating

> Communication is central to successful caring relationships and to effective team working. Listening is as important as what we say and do and essential for 'no decision about me without me'. Communication is the key to a good workplace with benefits for those in our care and staff alike. (Commissioning Board Chief Nursing Officer and DH Chief Nursing Adviser 2012: 13)

Whether it be 'mindfulness' (Chapter 5) or 'interprofessional education' (Chapter 8), Banja's (2010) 'normalisation of deviance' (Chapter 3) or 'reflection' (Chapter 7), each one of the chapters in this book places effective and compassionate communication as central to the health and social care practitioner's work.

For the purposes of a book on coping and thriving, the more we communicate with colleagues from all professional groups about our experiences in healthcare, the stronger the voice for change will become.

Last Thoughts

At the start of this chapter, we heard Robert's voice asserting clearly what he wanted from health and social care practitioners. Providing good-quality care is more than just getting the physical interventions right, however important they may be. If the practitioner is downtrodden, passive and demoralised, this adversely impacts on the person receiving care, therefore the demeanour of the practitioner is important.

One of the therapeutic factors in group work is what Yalom (2005) termed 'universality'. Universality was described as the experience within a group of realising that one is not alone in one's own problems, and that others have similar problems, concerns and anxieties.

In the Introduction to this book, I described a practitioner whom I called Cleo. In conversations with other practitioners like Cleo, there seemed to be a lack of opportunity to share experiences of health and social care in a constructive forum. In consequence, many practitioners appeared to be supressing emotions in an unhealthy way in order to maintain a professional facade when in patient environments.

With Yalom's concept of universality in mind, we hope that through reading this book, you have found some shared experience with other health and social care practitioners. We hope that you also feel that you have a toolkit to cope *and* thrive in the health and social care services today.

References

Ballatt, J. and Campling, P. (2011) *Intelligent Kindness*. London: Royal College of Psychiatrists.

Banja, J. (2010) 'The normalization of deviance in healthcare delivery', *Business Horizons*, 53 (2): 139.

Brookfield, S. (1995) *Becoming a Critically Reflective Teacher*. San Francisco, CA: Jossey-Bass.

Business Directory (2017) 'Social sustainability'. Available at: www.businessdictionary.com/ definition/social-sustainability.html (accessed 18 December 2017).

Carlson, K. (2017) *Nurses as Disrupters of Change*. Available at: www.ausmed.com/articles/ nurses-as-disrupters-agents-of-change/ (accessed September 2017).

Commissioning Board Chief Nursing Officer and Department of Health (DH) Chief Nursing Adviser (2012) *Compassion in Practice*. Leeds: DH.

Francis, R. (2013) *Report of the Mid Staffordshire NHS Foundation Trust Public Inquiry (The Francis Report): Executive Summary*. London: The Stationery Office.

Harris, R. (2006) 'Embracing your demons: An overview of acceptance and commitment ther-apy', *Psychotherapy in Australia, 12* (4): 2–8.

Hochschild, A.R. (1983) *The Managed Heart: Commercialisation of Human Feeling.* Berkeley, CA: University of California Press.

Mueller, J. (2017) *Creative Change.* Boston, MA: Houghton Mifflin Harcourt.

NHS (2017) Available at: www.nhs.uk/Conditions/stress-anxiety-depression/Pages/Time-management-tips.aspx (accessed December 2017).

Nursing and Midwifery Council (NMC) (2010) *Standards for Pre-registration Nurse Education.* London: NMC.

NMC (2017) *The NMC Register*, 30 September. London: NMC.

Oxford English Dictionary (OED) (2011) *Concise Oxford English Dictionary.* Oxford: Oxford University Press.

Rotter, J.B. (1954) *Social Learning and Clinical Psychology.* New York: Prentice-Hall.

Schön, D.A. (1983) *The Reflective Practitioner.* San Francisco, CA: Jossey-Bass.

Schön, D.A. (1987) *Educating the Reflective Practitioner: Toward a New Design for Teaching and Learning in the Professions.* San Francisco, CA: Jossey-Bass.

Storey, J. and Holti, R. (2013) *Towards a New Model of Leadership for the NHS.* London: NHS Leadership Academy.

Syed, M. (2016) *Black Box Thinking: Marginal Gains and the Secrets of High Performance.* London: John Murray.

Toffler, A. (1970) *Future Shock.* New York: Bantam Books.

Windle, G. (2011) 'What is resilience? A review and concept analysis', *Reviews in Clinical Gerontology, 21*: 152–69.

Yalom, I. (2005) *The Theory and Practice of Group Psychotherapy*, 5th edn. Cambridge, MA: Basic Books.

Index

6Cs 'Compassion in Practice' 16, 37, 38, 49, 135